WHY MEDICINE GOT SICK

ANATOMY OF A MODEL THAT HOLLOWED OUT HEALTH — AND IS NOW REINVENTING ITSELF

J. FRANCO

Health Shift

First edition published in 2025

Get in touch: contato@healthshift.com.br

www.porqueamedicinaadoeceu.com.br

TABLE OF CONTENTS

LETTER TO THE READER

This book was born out of unease—out of discomfort with how we deliver "healthcare" given our possibilities, available technology, and knowledge. The system has become a fragmented giant where professionals focus on organs instead of complex systems. Clinicians cling to protocols, patients cling to lab reports, and somewhere in the middle we lost sight of the whole.

Health is, by nature, a complex, transdisciplinary puzzle. Yet we keep trying to treat each piece in isolation, as if human beings were a bundle of disconnected parts. This book isn't about one specialty. It's about everything that shapes health—and how to reorganize care in a rational, effective way that can truly change a dangerous global trend toward illness. It's about where the forces that affect our health converge—and how technology is about to disrupt—and reorganize—all of it.

My story isn't that of a physician. I come from communications, marketing, technology, innovation, and the study of human behavior. But I've been on the other side, too. I've felt the chill of a hospital, the rush of a consultation, and the silence of an exhausted professional with neither time—nor scope—to genuinely listen and understand what affects the health of the person in front of them.

Over the years, I've seen up close how emotions shape the health of those around me—even when no doctor asked about them. I noticed the body is always signaling—and through a lot of research, I came to understand how deeply connected it is, how it's a machine of regeneration. It offers clues that today's procedures and protocols almost always ignore—clues that could be the key to faster diagnoses, treatments that truly work, and, ultimately, a population that falls ill less often.

I've lived all this as a curious mind—passionate about complex problems, data, science, psychology, and the design of services and solutions—and, above all, about the magic that happens when all those strands come together to change reality. Like many people, I simply don't accept that "taking care of health" is a synonym for "fixing what already broke," nor that, with all the possibilities of AI and validated technologies, healthcare should be content to act only after something goes wrong—without any commitment to the patient's potential for health.

Medicine that only corrects—necessary as it is—fails. It fails through inertia, omission, and lack of systemic vision. Caring for a life means recognizing that prevention isn't an "extra," it's the foundation. And that there is a great deal of science which must be woven into the healthcare ecosystem if we are to treat disease far more effectively.

That's why this book exists. Here, we'll traverse multiple disciplines, analyze real cases, and explore emerging technologies—because health demands exactly that: thinking that embraces complexity while remaining practical.

The concept of "adherence" (or engagement) and the methods for building transformative solutions will be crucial in this journey, but the focus of this first book is what comes before: the foundations—and the crises—of today's healthcare. No technology, however promising, will change our disastrous statistics if people don't use it, or if it isn't built to genuinely create better conditions for health. No solution is truly human if it doesn't recognize that health doesn't begin in a hospital or clinic, but in our daily lives, our choices, and our context.

At heart, this is a work about everything that permeates care—about how we can, and must, redesign how we treat the human body using intelligence, empathy, and a vision that crosses the borders of knowledge and puts them in order.

To get there, we face two rarely discussed obstacles. The first is almost a trick of the mind: our difficulty investing in what doesn't hurt yet. Taking care of ourselves to prevent disease wins no medals, earns no applause, and often delivers no immediately felt effect. The return is invisible. You prevent—and nothing happens. Paradoxically, that "nothing" is the greatest victory there is. The problem is, our brains aren't wired to value the absence of a problem—they want the solution to the problem that already exists. That's why getting people engaged in prevention is so hard.

The second obstacle is the system's very structure: protocolized dynamics built for the acute, the urgent, the easily measurable.

This book starts from the premise that transformation has to happen precisely in the gap—between the absence of symptoms and the search for meaning. And it will only be possible if we understand health as a phenomenon in which emotions, environment, diet, behavior, and bonds silently mold our bodies and our future. Most important of all: what to do with that understanding.

There is no such thing as "nothing" in prevention. There is an invisible process of construction—one that only becomes painfully visible when it's already too late. Our job is to flip that script. It's no accident that what began as a single-book project grew into a series—of which this is the first stand-alone volume. To tackle a topic this vast and full of traps—and to name the elephant in the healthcare room—I had to take two, three, four steps back in order to move forward. Because innovation doesn't start with technology. If we're to build new tools and services with the power to reverse the disastrous curves toward which global health is headed, we must critically revisit premises, situations, practices, and bodies of knowledge that rarely speak to each other.

Across the coming pages, you'll find ideas, provocations, data, essays, and case studies—and a sincere attempt to shine light on crucial blind spots: the intersections among fields of knowledge that barely converse. Consider this book an invitation—to think together, to question, to rebuild. And if I dare to write it, it isn't because I have all the answers, but because I'm fascinated by the right questions and by transdisciplinarity—where the real magic happens. And because I know I can help organize complex problems that deserve to be rethought.

If you're reading this, you're also seeking something more—whether you're a patient wanting more autonomy and more resolutive care; a health professional in search of more human practice; a student who needs a broader lens and knows AI will change everything; a manager looking for a more efficient system; or an entrepreneur focused on creating solutions that matter.

I'll consider this effort deeply worthwhile if I can show you even a little of the beauty and power that live at the frontiers of health knowledge—and the scale of the historical opportunity before us. And, of course, if a few lights switch on for you.

See you between the lines.

João Franco.

INTRODUCTION

First things first: **what is health**?

Most people hesitate before answering. Even among healthcare professionals, healthtech CEOs, policymakers, and physicians, what you usually hear is vague, defensive, or simply wrong.

The way we practice health today is built on a statistical abstraction — a number that stays "within range," a test that comes back "normal." But the absence of a symptom has never guaranteed vitality. We live in a troubling paradox: the more sensors, algorithms, and clinical protocols we create, the faster chronic diseases spread, anxiety escalates, and burnout becomes institutionalized as one of the defining syndromes of our time.

Technology has evolved. Care hasn't kept up. We continue treating illness only after it has won, tracking risks we don't fully understand, reacting to symptoms as though they existed without context, history, cause, or meaning.

This book is born from the urgency to dismantle that model — not to attack medicine, but to rebuild it from its core outward. It's an invitation to rethink what it means to be healthy, to care, to prevent, to heal — and to challenge everything we've misunderstood along the way.

You'll understand why digital health often fails, even when built with good intentions. You'll see how emotions, habits, environment, algorithms, and biochemistry are not isolated forces but parts of one living system. You'll recognize how fragmentation — between disciplines, between professionals, between truths — erodes the very potential of care. And you'll gain access to tangible, innovative proposals that reimagine health as an **intelligent, integrated system designed to sustain life**.

Because the future of health will be transversal, emotional, continuous, and regenerative. It demands a **new pact** — between those who care, those who are cared for, those who design systems, and those who live within them.

This book is about what happens when care regains its meaning — yes, with technology, but above all with a **new logic**. And it's about everything already underway to make that transformation real.

CHAPTER 1
ABSENCE OF SYMPTOMS IS NOT HEALTH

THE ORIGINS OF HEALTH DEFINED AS THE ABSENCE OF DISEASE

From Antiquity to the present day, health has remained an elusive and misunderstood concept. The reductionist view that equates health merely with the absence of physical symptoms has deep roots; it was constructed throughout the history of Western medicine and eventually entrenched itself as a silent paradigm, institutionally reinforced over time. This definition ignores the profound complexity involved in the experience of living truly healthily. It is a fundamental conceptual error with deep roots, tracing back to the philosophical and scientific foundations of medicine itself—from Hippocrates and Galen to the development of modern medical practices and clinical specializations.

For centuries, medicine has organized itself around the ailing body, not the healthy one. Even the Hippocratic Oath leaned more heavily toward curing infirmity than maintaining or enhancing integral health. The first Western medical schools, founded under Greco-Roman influence, emphasized symptoms as the focal point of diagnosis and treatment. Health was thus identified as the direct opposite of disease—a concept defined by negation and reaction. This paradigm became deeply ingrained, transforming medicine into a practice focused neither on prevention nor regeneration.

In the 17th century, René Descartes' proposed mind-body dualism further solidified this mindset. The body became a machine comprised of parts that could fail and, if so, required repair. This fragmented model stifled the broader understanding of health preserved by traditions such as Ayurveda and Traditional Chinese Medicine, which viewed health as an equilibrium between body, emotions, environment, and relationships.

The Industrial Revolution deepened this mechanistic logic by instilling an obsession with productivity and efficiency into medical practice. Physicians began to be trained almost exclusively to identify and eliminate symptoms rapidly, with little room to consider emotional, social, or environmental variables. Consequently, health institutions began to operate based on the absence of disease. This molded hospitals, clinics, and universities according to a corrective and emergency-driven logic. Since then, any physical or emotional deviation from the norm has been immediately interpreted as illness or pre-illness, rather than a potentially healthy or adaptive signal warranting analysis.

In the 20th century, accelerated industrialization and the rise of major pharmaceutical companies further entrenched the absence of symptoms as the definitive criterion for health, becoming part of the dominant commercial standard. A model based on constant medicalization and routine pharmacological intervention took hold, transforming often natural and transient symptoms into clinical conditions requiring medication. The advent of laboratory testing and imaging—despite being significant technological breakthroughs—ultimately reinforced this symptomatic paradigm. Small bodily alterations began to be treated with drugs, creating a younger population that is increasingly medicated yet rarely living at its full health potential.

This simplification also found fertile ground in the logic of late-stage capitalism (from the 1970s onward), which introduced market and performance dynamics into healthcare. It spawned a multi-billion dollar industry focused exclusively on the continuous treatment of disease, selling a sensation of well-being encapsulated in often unnecessary medications and procedures. Health ceased to be intrinsic and became a product, dependent on the elimination of symptoms measurable in disconnected routine clinical exams.

However, vigorous critiques of this reductionist paradigm began to emerge in the mid-20th century. In 1946, the World Health Organization (WHO) presented a definition of health that was groundbreaking for its time, though frequently ignored in daily clinical practice: "Health is a state of complete physical, mental and social well-being and not merely the absence of disease or infirmity." Even so, the reality of healthcare rarely caught up with this expanded vision. The system remained trapped in a clinical operation based on symptomatic elimination, far removed from the holistic approach proposed by the WHO nearly a century ago.

In parallel, prominent 20th-century theorists like Aaron Antonovsky proposed conceptual alternatives, such as the salutogenic model. Unlike the prevailing pathogenic paradigm, the salutogenic model emphasizes the origins and development of health. It suggests that people are naturally inclined to feel well, provided their environment, emotions, and relationships are positive. Antonovsky believed medicine should focus on identifying and promoting these health factors, rather than concentrating solely on curing disease.

More recently, at the turn of the 21st century, positive psychology deepened this critique. Studies by Martin Seligman (Authentic Happiness Theory) and Mihaly Csikszentmihalyi (Flow Theory) opened a new chapter in the discussion on positive health. It invites us to view health beyond the mere absence of disease, highlighting the importance of thriving and achieving high levels of emotional, physical, and social well-being, both individually and collectively. Many classified as "healthy" by traditional medicine were, in practice, living with critically low levels of purpose, connection, and vitality. This field of research helped expose what many had long intuited but few institutions recognized: true health begins where exams end; it is movement, adaptation, and the continuous expression of life.

Yet, this limited vision has shaped an entire ecosystem of "care" that treats the individual superficially, reacting only to what is visible, perceptible, and measurable. In this dominant model, symptoms are viewed as adversaries to be swiftly eliminated, rather than recognized as vital signals revealing the internal and external context in which an individual is situated. This approach restricts our understanding of the human body and hollows out the deepest meaning of health: the vital potency of the human being.

SYMPTOM-BASED MEDICINE AND THE HOLLOWING OUT OF VITAL POTENCY

In his classic work *The Normal and the Pathological*, philosopher and physician Georges Canguilhem warned of the dangers of this simplification, suggesting that symptoms should not be treated as isolated signs, but as complex, adaptive manifestations of the human body in response to environmental adversity. For Canguilhem, an individual can be considered truly healthy when they can adapt and respond to constant internal and external changes with vigor, efficiency, and emotional balance—distinct from a mechanistic view of adaptation. He proposes a vision that inverts the traditional paradigm: health is not the absence of suffering or pathology, but the presence of a creative and resilient capacity for adaptation.

Here, a distinction is necessary: not all adaptation favors health. The author suggests we possess an innate capacity to adapt to life's challenges —a continuous negotiation between body and environment that causes physiological changes—and this is a sign of health. However, we must be vigilant: in an environment with chronically adverse conditions, this adaptation, if misunderstood, can expose the individual to a "toxic adaptability" that allows for survival but at a high cost, ultimately working against their health.

Science is beginning to strongly support this perspective. Recent studies in neurobiology and psychosomatics have robustly revealed that the human body frequently generates symptoms as adaptive, necessary responses to challenging life contexts or significant environmental changes. For instance, a moderate inflammatory response—frequently treated by traditional medicine as a symptom to be rapidly suppressed by medication—is often a healthy, adaptive biological strategy to heal and protect the body from further damage, and it warrants investigation. Researchers such as neuroscientist Antonio Damasio, author of the renowned book *Descartes' Error*, clearly demonstrate that separating physical symptoms from emotional and social contexts is scientifically incorrect and clinically imprecise.

Conventional medicine still relies on treating isolated symptoms without considering the systemic complexity of human health. This is particularly evident in modern chronic diseases such as hypertension, type 2 diabetes, metabolic syndrome, and various autoimmune conditions. In these cases, the traditional approach focuses on reducing biometric levels like glucose, cholesterol, or blood pressure, treating these numbers as if they were the sole indicators of health or disease. But these data points are merely the visible tips of a deep iceberg, which includes lifestyle, stress, isolation, and a lack of purpose.

One of the most explicit examples of this draining of meaning is the widespread medicalization of emotions, especially anxiety and sadness, which often require responses and reactions at the level of environment and living conditions. In recent decades, the expansion of psychiatric diagnoses has led to a scenario where millions are treated for emotions that are, in fact, part of life or even essential to it. Psychiatric medications are prescribed on a massive scale, often as the only solution, without considering life context, interpersonal relationships, the emotional significance of symptoms, or the need for deeper lifestyle changes. In 2018, a study published in the prestigious medical journal *The Lancet* issued a warning about what it described as the "silent epidemic of the medicalization of life." The study clearly highlighted the dangers of a model that focuses excessively on isolated symptoms and the potential harm this causes to collective health today.

Imagine a scenario where symptoms are pieces of an unfinished puzzle—each revealing an aspect of our health. When we treat these symptoms as obstacles to be quickly eliminated without investigating their roots, we sow a silent mistrust within ourselves. It begins to feel as though our body is constantly under attack, incapable of healing or adapting on its own. This approach leads us into a continuous dependency on medical treatments, which often only mask the true emotions or existential issues originating the symptoms. In this dominant dynamic, our innate ability to regenerate and adapt to the world becomes invisible and even discredited by the very medicine that should be its ally.

Recent research conducted by institutions like Harvard Medical

School and Stanford has provided compelling evidence of this phenomenon. In a study led by Professor Bruce McEwen's team, it became evident that constant exposure to the idea of illness and fragility intensifies patients' physiological and emotional vulnerability. This triggers chronic states of stress that, surprisingly, increase the risk of developing disease. Curiously, the traditional medical model, focused on treating symptoms, may actually diminish people's integral health.

This critique does not seek to invalidate the importance of conventional medical treatment in cases of severe or urgent symptoms. On the contrary: what is proposed is a broadening of vision. Symptoms must be understood as signals of broader imbalances that demand listening and reconnection. 21st-century medicine can no longer operate under the simple, superficial logic of rapidly eliminating visible symptoms; it must assume the role of a conscious interpreter of these signals, treating them at their deepest, most integrative causes and returning agency over life to the patient.

Studies in cognitive neuroscience and complexity sciences, such as those by Francisco Varela and Humberto Maturana on embodied cognition, have also offered important tools for reconnecting health and vital potency. They argue that health cannot be measured by the silence of symptoms, but by the capacity for self-organization in the face of life's flow. And no exam, however modern, is capable of capturing this dimension alone.

THE CONSEQUENCES OF A REDUCTIONIST MODEL

Adopting this fragmented model of medicine has practical repercussions that cut deep into the entire healthcare system and compromise the care provided. By reducing health to the elimination of detectable symptoms or the spot-correction of clinical deviations, we have created a system that prioritizes standardized procedures over the true promotion of integral health. This inversion of priorities generates immense costs for society.

One of the most visible consequences of this paradigm is the intense medicalization of daily life. Situations that could be managed with simple lifestyle changes, qualified listening, or adequate psychosocial support end up being treated essentially with indiscriminately prescribed medications. Many medical prescriptions in the Western world could be replaced by non-pharmacological interventions, offering superior results and fewer side effects. But the fragmented system and the culture of immediacy breed a medical environment that values the speed of symptom relief over the true resolution of root causes.

Another profound impact of this model is the exponential rise in unnecessary medical interventions. The phenomenon known as *overdiagnosis*, detailed by Australian physician and researcher Alexandra Barratt, exposes how the obsession with early diagnosis and immediate intervention can cause more harm than good. Screenings such as annual mammograms in young women, PSA tests in low-risk populations, or the indiscriminate use of CT scans and MRIs for common lower back pain fuel a cycle of misdiagnosis, aggressive treatments, and avoidable sequelae. And, to make matters worse, there is little structure in place to actually influence the root cause of what is found.

These excessive interventions place dangerous pressure on already overburdened health systems. Data published by the *Journal of the American Medical Association* indicates that up to 25% of healthcare spending in the United States is related to procedures or treatments considered useless or unnecessary. In Brazil, according to the Institute of Supplemental Health Studies, approximately 15% of costs in the private health sector are associated with waste, including unnecessary procedures. We are talking about billions of dollars invested every year in misguided approaches, while integral prevention initiatives—based on healthy nutrition, physical activity, emotional support, and effective community practices—remain underfunded and neglected.

When immediate quantitative indicators are prioritized, such as temporary symptom reduction or the volume of procedures performed, many managers fail to invest in structural transformations like health education, healthy cities, social infrastructure, and cultural changes. The result is a vicious cycle where the most vulnerable populations remain trapped in episodic treatments and frequent returns to emergency rooms, without access to resources that could promote lasting health.

And it doesn't stop there. This fragmented view also contributes to the alarming rise in chronic diseases. The traditional biomedical model, which prioritizes acute and immediate responses, systematically fails to deal with the complexity of these conditions, which require continuous monitoring, personalization, patient education, and profound habit changes. It is no coincidence that diseases like diabetes, obesity, hypertension, and emotional disorders have become global epidemics. The lack of a truly integrative and preventive approach has allowed these problems to multiply silently, revealing a scenario where billions of people live with conditions that could have been avoided or mitigated. Curiously, "healthcare" does not include an incisive look at what actually affects health.

By neglecting the broader context of people's lives, this medical approach has weakened the bond between healthcare professionals and patients. The logic of productivity, rigid protocols, and the culture of clocked appointments has dehumanized clinical care. Studies from Harvard Medical School indicate that physicians frequently express frustration and professional burnout due to productivity pressures and the reduction of time dedicated to listening to and understanding the patient in their totality. This loss harms the professional as well, creating an environment that generates chronic frustration, potentially leading to medical errors and diminishing the overall efficacy of treatments.

This scenario contributes to a growing disconnection between individuals and their own bodies, reinforcing the idea that health must be administered exclusively by experts. Consequently, people lose confidence in their capacity to recognize signs, interpret sensations, and make conscious decisions about their well-being.

This alienation from one's own body is worrying because it distances the individual from active participation in their health, resulting in continuous dependence on medical services even for trivial matters. By recognizing this impasse, we open space for a new, more pragmatic, lucid, and human perspective on what it truly means to promote health, sustain care, and regenerate lives. It is this perspective that we will begin to build, step by step, throughout this work.

THEMATIC FOCUS: THE CONSEQUENCES OF REDUCTIONIST MEDICINE

Economic Impact

- High spending on avoidable procedures
- Overburdening of public systems
- Underfunding of preventive actions

Social Impact

- Excessive medicalization of daily life
- Weakening of community bonds
- Widening of health inequalities

Individual Impact

- Alienation of individuals from their own bodies
- Continuous dependence on medical services
- Loss of autonomy over personal decisions

THE RISK OF SHALLOW METRICS

Reducing health to the absence of symptoms presumes they are always evident. This conceals a dangerous reality: many silent conditions remain invisible when health is defined by the lack of perceptible manifestations. This view generates metrics that are easy to interpret but too shallow to reflect the true state of an individual's health.

LDL cholesterol, known as "bad cholesterol," is widely used in routine laboratory exams as an essential metric for cardiovascular health. While useful, focusing exclusively on this marker ignores critical nuances. Recent studies, such as those from Harvard Medical School published in the *Journal of the American College of Cardiology*, show that people with LDL levels considered "normal" may still be at high cardiovascular risk due to hidden factors like chronic inflammation, insulin resistance, or alterations in the lipoprotein particle profile. In such cases, statistical "normality" masks clinical instability.

The classic assessment of fasting glucose, used in type 2 diabetes prevention, follows this same logic. While useful, it disregards important variations such as post-meal glycemic spikes and daily glycemic stability. Studies show that individuals with "normal" fasting glucose may present inflammatory fluctuations after meals, associated with significant metabolic risks (Zeevi et al., 2015; *Cell Metabolism*). Often, the fasting duration itself is inadequate for the exam (a 12-hour fast can mask imbalances, yet it is not uncommon for professionals to allow this test alongside others requiring different fasting times). Appearing normal on paper does not equate to being metabolically protected.

THEMATIC FOCUS: SHALLOW INDICATORS VS. DEEP INDICATORS

Isolated LDL

→ Complete lipoprotein profile and inflammatory status

Fasting Glucose

→ Continuous monitoring and daily glycemic stability

BMI (Body Mass Index)

→ Detailed body composition and visceral fat percentage

Simple Mental Health Questionnaires

→ Complete neuropsychological evaluation and qualitative analysis of emotional symptoms

Spot Blood Pressure

→ Blood pressure variability and stress response

Single Renal Function Test (Isolated Creatinine)

→ Evaluation of renal function along the time and early damage markers

When test results fall within population averages, both physicians and patients tend to become complacent. The phrase "everything looks normal" sounds reassuring, yet it frequently disarms critical judgment and sabotages interventions that could be decisive. It creates resistance to change at the precise moment when change is still light, achievable, and accessible. Furthermore, it reinforces a reactive model: as long as the numbers appear acceptable, no one investigates what remains silent, and preventive measures are left untaken. It is only when symptoms become acute that a race against time begins, resulting in a clinical cycle that merely reacts. And when it finally responds, it is often too late, more expensive, and more painful. This is a point of absolute interest to the patient, yet it is clearly marginalized in medical education and clinical practice.

To illustrate the risk of this approach, one need only look at autoimmune diseases. Research from the National Institutes of Health (UK) shows that patients often spend years battling vague symptoms such as fatigue, diffuse pain, and emotional shifts without a clear diagnosis, simply because traditional exams remain "normal." This "illusory normality" delays crucial diagnoses, prolongs suffering, and amplifies often irreversible damage to the body, particularly in diseases like lupus or rheumatoid arthritis.

The same applies to mental health. The use of generic questionnaires and standardized metrics to evaluate depression or anxiety ignores the emotional, cultural, and contextual nuances of the human experience. Many individuals with anxiety symptoms do not exhibit the typical signs required by official diagnostic criteria, and thus remain invisible or poorly managed within the current clinical system.

The absence of apparent disease cannot be treated as a finish line, but rather as a starting point for a deeper, continuous investigation into the integral state of health. More sensitive tools, such as heart rate variability (HRV), systemic inflammation levels (like ultra-sensitive C-reactive protein), or functional assessments of the gut microbiota, are emerging as key allies in detecting risks before symptoms become visible (Harvard School of Public Health, 2023).

It is fundamental to promote a paradigm shift in how we understand what it means to be healthy. Health is movement, plasticity, coherence, and context. This requires stepping out of the logic of delayed response and investing in a genuinely proactive clinical mindset that unites advanced analytics, predictive algorithms, artificial intelligence, and, above all, a refined clinical listening committed to what is not instantly revealed by basic exams. Normality must stop acting as an anesthetic. It needs to start acting as a catalyst.

RETHINKING THE ESSENCE OF HEALTH

Broadening our vision of health requires breaking with traditional paradigms that have dominated the discourse of healthcare institutions and solutions for decades. It is about making tangible, in practice, mechanisms that promote health as an integral potency, leveraging the opportunities generated by the explosion of artificial intelligence and the Internet of Things (IoT). However, this will not happen automatically, nor will it happen if we remain anchored to simplistic premises of what it means to care for one's health. An optimal state of health implies the full functioning of an individual's physical, emotional, cognitive, and social capacities—capabilities that are increasingly taxed in a daily life incalculably more hectic than it was a few hundred years ago (and even more so than just a few years ago). In other words, health ceases to be a defensive stance against disease and becomes an offensive attitude toward vitality, potency, and well-being.

This shift is strongly inspired by the biopsychosocial model proposed by George Engel in the 1970s, which considers the interaction between biological, psychological, and social factors in understanding health and disease. However, the current approach broadens these foundations by incorporating the data and technological tools accessible to us today.

In the case of depression, beyond chemical alterations in the brain that may even be caused by nutrient deficiency (biological factor), it is fundamental to consider emotional aspects, such as trauma and stress (psychological factor), as well as the environment in which the person lives, including their family relationships and socioeconomic conditions (social factor). Similarly, in chronic diseases like diabetes, disease control involves medication (biological), but also stress management and motivation for treatment adherence (psychological), alongside family support and access to adequate health services (social).

Engel warned long ago that health could not be understood simply as the absence of physical disease. It was necessary to concretely integrate the psychological and social factors that shape the human experience. This is not new. Yet, even after more than four decades, the dominant clinical discourse still ignores or drastically minimizes these factors.

For this transformation to occur, health needs to be constantly monitored and strengthened using more sensitive parameters that detect functions and resources—bodily, emotional, and social—long before evident pathologies emerge.

A concrete and highly effective example is the use of sensitive biomarkers of biological aging. Among them are telomeres—structures located at the ends of chromosomes that function as "protective caps" for genetic material.

As we age, telomeres shorten, serving as indicators of cellular wear over time. Another relevant marker is epigenetic indices, such as "Horvath's clock," based on chemical modifications to DNA known as methylation. These modifications do not alter the genetic sequence but influence how genes are expressed, allowing for an estimation of the organism's biological age, which may be higher or lower than chronological age depending on factors like lifestyle and environment.

Furthermore, continuous measurements of cardiorespiratory capacity, such as VO2 max, evaluate the maximum amount of oxygen the body can utilize during intense physical activity and directly reflect the functional integrity of the heart, lungs, and muscles. These indicators offer a powerful, early view of physiological status, unlike traditional medicine, which reacts only after damage has set in. Based on these markers, health professionals can guide proactive and personalized strategies.

The ideal scenario involves a new mindset that understands health as a permanent investment in human potency. This requires incorporating technologies like artificial intelligence and machine learning to detect early patterns of functional loss and risk, allowing for interventions before symptoms manifest. It is about refusing to stand idly by while problems take root and vitality is lost, instead acting beneficially for the patient before bodily imbalance becomes established. In this model, technology and humanization cease to be opposing extremes and become a complementary ecosystem dedicated to the continuous construction of vital potency.

By viewing each patient as an integral being in process, full of capacities and potential, we also recover the humanizing role of the health professional as an agent of transformation capable of awakening the best in others, with a purpose aligned with what healthcare can and should be in the 21st century.

STUDIES CHALLENGING THE "NORMAL" EXAM RESULT

The authority of laboratory exams in modern clinical practice rests on a tripod: standardization, statistics, and replicability. But as medicine advances to understand health as a dynamic, multifactorial, and individualized process, this tripod begins to wobble. A growing body of scientific literature is showing that parameters "within normal range" can hide relevant pathological processes, especially in the early stages of imbalance or in cases of functional disease, which challenge the binary logic of "healthy vs. sick."

At insulin levels between 7 and 9 µU/mL—a range widely accepted as "okay"—there is a higher incidence of visceral fat gain, hepatic alterations, and post-meal fatigue. These manifestations are early indications of so-called "functional metabolic disease," still invisible to the traditional clinical eye.

The advance of functional and integrative medicine is reigniting the urgency for a contextualized analysis of biomarkers. The evaluation of salivary cortisol at different times of the day better detects imbalances in the HPA axis (hypothalamus–pituitary–adrenal), which regulates stress, metabolism, the immune system, and hormonal balance. Curiously, these imbalances often go unnoticed in conventional serum cortisol exams, which capture only a single moment in the day.

The critique also extends to the inflammatory marker CRP (C-

Reactive Protein). Values up to 3 mg/L are considered "normal," but research by the American Heart Association shows that levels between 2 and 3 mg/L are already associated with low-grade chronic inflammation and higher cardiovascular risk. In at-risk populations, this is often the beginning of silent illness, yet it remains ignored by current protocols.

In psychiatry, the use of biological markers such as folic acid, vitamin D, and magnesium to evaluate depressive or anxious states still meets resistance in orthodox psychiatry, despite various specialists and studies—such as those published in the *Journal of Affective Disorders*—associating low (yet technically "normal") levels of these substances with chronic fatigue, insomnia, loss of libido, and attention deficits.

Liver function tests follow the same pattern: AST and ALT enzymes, used to monitor liver inflammation, vary between laboratories and frequently minimize mild increases labeled as normal, even when signs of hepatic steatosis, inflammation, or toxicity are present. A study in *Hepatology International* showed that more than 40% of patients diagnosed with NASH (non-alcoholic steatohepatitis) had ALT levels within the normal range in exams taken the previous year.

Various groups of health professionals are taking a stronger stand on the inadequacy of current laboratory standards. The American Association of Clinical Endocrinologists proposed as early as 2003 revising the TSH normality range to between 0.3 and 2.5, rather than the previously usual 0.4 – 4.5. Other entities, such as the Endocrine Society and the American College of Cardiology, have released guidelines recognizing the need to evaluate the "functional normal."

The critique extends to the very process of constructing reference tables. Many are based on population samples that do not exclude individuals with silent pathologies, metabolic disorders, or those on medication. A study in *Clinical Biochemistry* revealed that in several North American laboratories, reference values for liver and kidney markers were based on mixed cohorts without filters for metabolic health or inflammatory status. This directly compromises the sensitivity of standard ranges.

This distortion is aggravated when applied to populations with specific physiological parameters. Children, the elderly, menopausal women, athletes, neurodivergent individuals, and so on, present metabolisms and physiological parameters that do not always align with population average tables. And here, a gentle reminder is in order: averages do not exist in reality; they are abstract numbers resulting from a mathematical operation. Imagine two adult men with a height of 1.80m. What if I tell you that they weigh, on average, 85kg? Nothing noteworthy, right? But what if I tell you that to compose this average, we have one man weighing 35kg and another weighing 135kg? The average, on its own, does not reflect reality—by definition. Despite being an obvious fact, in practice, it is frequently ignored.

Exams that combine different markers into functional panels are proving more effective. The Dutch Test for urinary hormone analysis, organic acid panels for metabolic mapping, and continuous glucose monitors are examples that allow for more contextual, dynamic, and integrated readings, without relying exclusively on universal ranges.

And what does "normal" mean in a significantly ailing world? When the population average is hypertensive, anxious, obese, and suffering from fragmented sleep, taking its parameters as a reference for health is, at the very least, an exercise in technical cynicism. As epidemiologist Geoffrey Rose points out, "the definition of normality as a population average condemns us to normalize pathology."

This discussion inevitably leads us to the need to review not only reference ranges but also the criteria by which we decide what merits intervention. There are cases where minimal variations, even without exceeding limits, are already associated with real symptoms, loss of functionality, and reduced vitality. The exam doesn't lie. But a shallow reading does.

Therefore, the movement to update reference tables must be seen as an ethical imperative. Just as medicine updates its clinical protocols based on new evidence, laboratory values must also keep pace with discoveries in physiology, biochemistry, and integrative clinical practice. The model of normality, like any marker, must be an open hypothesis.

PERSPECTIVES FOR A FUTURE THAT SEES LESS EVIDENT SYMPTOMS

Some advanced research centers, such as the Institute for Functional Medicine (USA), are already adopting models based on integrated maps of symptoms, life history, dietary style, exposure to environmental toxins, trauma, and genetic predisposition. The goal is to construct a risk reading—a kind of vulnerability profile that allows the clinician to intervene earlier.

This type of approach is already showing results in specific contexts. In patients with autoimmune diseases, active listening to initial signs can anticipate inflammatory flare-ups. The earliest health "data" is often a sensation. Trained clinical intuition, combined with relationship-oriented technology, can transform this sensation into predictive evidence. Patients who frequently report a "sensation of head pressure at the end of the day" or "shortness of breath even at mild rest," even with normal exams, should be evaluated with lenses that see dysfunction before disease. The medicine of the future begins in the body's physiological narrative.

In China, high-complexity integrative clinics are applying algorithms to scan subjective symptoms described on digital platforms, cross-referencing this data with tongue images, pulse variations, facial analysis, and body temperature, integrating principles of traditional Chinese medicine with machine learning. The proposal is to build a more sensitive clinical scope, oriented toward the organism's functional balance. It is a way of placing artificial intelligence at the service of the somatic intelligence the body already possesses, but which conventional clinical practice still does not know how to measure.

Another emerging axis is the use of digital health diaries: apps where patients report their daily experiences, emotional states, energy levels, and sleep quality. Projects like Bearable (UK) and Cara Care (Germany) have demonstrated predictive value: subtle changes in reporting patterns anticipate pain flare-ups, anxiety crises, and even glycemic fluctuations in patients with chronic diseases. This data, structured consistently, becomes legitimate and earlier clinical indicators.

It is crucial that this model of listening be digitized and interpreted with clinical care, as there is a risk of over-interpretation or the medicalization of "discomfort." Therefore, a professional capable of distinguishing between fleeting sensations and emerging patterns of dysfunction is necessary. When the professional recognizes that the patient perceives something before the exam does and values that perception, a partnership is created. This shift impacts even therapeutic adherence: patients who feel heard become active participants in their own care.

In practice, this means the check-up of the future goes beyond a battery of standardized tests to include a personalized investigation process that begins with deep listening. The exam, however sophisticated, is a snapshot. The relevant clinical question will not just be "what is the value?" but "what does this value mean for this person, at this point in their history?"

Functional and integrative medicine is already consolidating broader forms of laboratory interpretation. One of the most discussed is the distinction between reference values and optimal values. While the reference interval describes the statistical average of the tested population, the optimal range points to levels associated with full functional health: lower inflammation, greater hormonal stability, and superior cellular performance. This approach is already applied, with good results, to exams such as ferritin, vitamin D, B12, insulin, and TSH.

This distinction between "normal" and "healthy" needs to be communicated responsibly to the patient. This is expanded consciousness. Well-prepared doctors know how to strike this balance: they acknowledge the comfort that a "within standard" result can bring, but also explain that this does not necessarily mean physiological equilibrium. The exam needs to be translated. This clinical pedagogy is one of the pillars of prevention: when patients understand their own markers, they become agents of their health.

Digital platforms are already moving in this direction. Solutions like InsideTracker (USA) and startups like Carevolution (Europe) combine laboratory data, clinical history, and lifestyle habits to produce customized functional maps. Instead of simply displaying values, these tools suggest areas for early attention, adjustment strategies, and care proposals based on scientific evidence. The clinical intelligence of these platforms is still nascent, but they point the way: interpreting is more valuable than simply measuring.

Data must be integrated with the nuances of daily life. A slightly high TSH may be related to poor sleep. CRP can rise after acute stress or a mild infection. Urea can vary after an intense workout. Vitamin D oscillates with the season, location, skin tone, clothing habits, and work environment. Clinical interpretation needs to cross-reference science with sensitivity, statistics with humanity. And here enters the role of the algorithm architects, who are quite human and often thousands of miles away from those who will benefit (or not) from the innovation. Algorithms answer questions and follow paths defined by someone. In other words, to evolve in this integral vision, we need to ask good questions and orchestrate statistical and complex models capable of seeking answers where gaps currently exist.

In this sense, one of the most promising paths is the use of hybrid algorithms: built on artificial intelligence but supervised by experienced clinicians to produce "functional health panels" or rich outputs that consider contexts. Instead of returning a list of isolated markers to the patient, these platforms create narratives of risk and vitality, associating exams with reported symptoms, behavioral patterns, and medical history. Projects like FunctionIQ in Australia or the Personal Health Dashboard in Canada have tested this type of approach with good results in engagement, understanding, and therapeutic adherence.

Below, we present a panorama of global and Brazilian initiatives that are redefining the interpretation of laboratory exams by integrating technology, clinical listening, and subjective data.

THEMATIC FOCUS: INNOVATIVE INITIATIVES IN REINTERPRETING LABORATORY EXAMS

Ellipsis Health (USA)

- **Description:** A platform using AI to analyze speech patterns and detect early signs of mental distress in remote consultations.
- **Differentiators:** Analyzes intonation, pauses, and emotional vocabulary to complement human listening.
- **Impact:** Demonstrated over 80% accuracy in screening for mild depression cases that would go unnoticed on traditional scales.

Taliaz (Israel)

- **Description:** A healthtech firm crossing genetic data, behavioral patterns, and clinical history to suggest personalized approaches in mental health.
- **Differentiators:** Proposes strategies adjusted to patient individuality, based on expanded clinical intelligence.
- **Impact:** Reduced treatment response time and improved therapeutic adherence in patients with depression.

Ada Health (Germany)

- **Description:** An AI-supported symptom self-assessment app used by patients to identify ambiguous health patterns.
- **Differentiators:** Detailed questioning and deep listening to reported symptoms.
- **Impact:** Assisted in the early identification of conditions that did not constitute a diagnosable disease but merited clinical attention.

InsideTracker (USA)

- **Description:** A platform combining laboratory data, clinical history, and lifestyle habits to produce customized functional maps.
- **Differentiators:** Suggests areas for early attention and intervention strategies based on peer-reviewed scientific literature.
- **Impact:** Increased patient understanding of their own markers and encouraged positive lifestyle changes.

Carevolution (Europe)

- **Description:** A platform offering functional health panels, associating exams with reported symptoms and behavioral patterns.

- **Differentiators:** Uses AI supervised by experienced clinicians to create narratives of risk and vitality.
- **Impact:** Increased patient engagement and improved therapeutic adherence.

Functional Mind (USA)

- **Description:** An AI platform for functional medicine that analyzes patient data to automate root cause identification.
- **Differentiators:** Uses specialized AI, trained on scientific literature, to interpret exams and clinical notes.
- **Impact:** Reduces clinician analysis time, accelerates diagnoses, and facilitates the creation of personalized therapies.

HeartMath Institute (USA)

- **Description:** A research center studying heart rate variability (HRV) as an indicator of emotional and physiological health.
- **Differentiators:** Developed techniques to improve cardiac coherence and stress resilience.
- **Impact:** Demonstrated that coherent HRV patterns are associated with cardiovascular health, emotional resilience, and immunity.

OmniLAMP (Brazil)

- **Description:** A portable device performing molecular tests via RT-LAMP for infectious disease diagnosis.
- **Differentiators:** Does not require complex laboratory equipment.

- **Impact:** Received the Abril & Dasa Medical Innovation Award for its standout role in combating the COVID-19 pandemic.

CHAPTER 2
MEDICINE AS A RESPONSE TO DEATH

Astonishingly, modern medicine (and the entire rationale that dictates the dynamics of healthcare) was not born out of a love for life. It was born out of a fear of death. It is in this simple, uncomfortable clash that the root of the deepest Western medical contradiction lies: the Herculean effort to prolong lives while remaining content that these extended lives do not necessarily translate into lives lived well—a factor often outside its scope.

Historically, medicine has walked hand-in-hand with the persistent shadow of death. From its origins in classical antiquity, through the unsanitary corridors of medieval hospitals, to the sterilized rooms of modern clinics, it has evolved primarily as a response to the immediate threat of death, rather than a pathway for the active promotion of integral health. Although contemporary Western medicine likes to present itself as "evidence-based" and committed to "well-being," its history reveals otherwise: its central motivation always has been, and still is, to some extent, to fight the inevitable.

Hippocrates, often considered the "father of medicine," lived in times marked by devastating epidemics and a scarcity of doctors. The famous Hippocratic Oath, while containing the noble principle of "do no harm," implicitly reveals a greater preoccupation with imminent death than with the full flourishing of health. In Ancient Greece, a physician's worth was measured by their ability to intervene at the threshold between life and death.

This emergency-centric approach intensified during the European Middle Ages, a period when death was virtually omnipresent. Epidemics like the Black Death, which decimated a third of the European population in the 14th century, turned medicine into a desperate act. Physicians, often conflated with healers or priests, operated constantly under death's shadow, and the line between clinical care and spiritual comfort was thin. Cures were rare; fear was constant. The medieval hospital symbolizes this reactive medicine: it was for sheltering the dying and offering a less solitary end. The word "hospital" comes from the Latin *hospitium*—lodging, shelter. What was promised was minimal relief in the face of inevitable suffering.

Even the Renaissance, with its obsession with knowledge and anatomy, did not break this logic. Andreas Vesalius, the father of modern anatomy, revolutionized the study of the body with his work *De Humani Corporis Fabrica* (1543). Anatomical dissection was seen as a means of understanding established diseases, and medicine remained subservient to the logic of death, albeit now with more instruments and greater precision.

Philosophers of science and medical historians, such as Michel Foucault in his seminal *The Birth of the Clinic* (1963), reinforce this view. According to Foucault, the traditional medical gaze was born from and for death, with clinical practices that view the patient as an object to be saved, before being fully understood as a human being.

Research reveals that concepts like prevention, quality of life, and integral health only recently began to enter official guidelines. Even so, these areas remain underfunded and possess lower status when compared to the specialties that dominate the medical landscape.

The intention here is to clearly understand the structural obsession of the practice: immediate survival. Recognizing this origin allows us to grasp its historical limitations, and then to overcome them. Acknowledging that medicine was born as the *daughter of death* is the first step toward fundamentally rethinking its practical focus and scope, enabling it to evolve with less friction in the face of all that technology will provide and the new, horizontalized "specialties" that connect the many parts defining a person's health.

EMERGENCY MEDICINE AND THE TRADITION OF REACTION

Emergency medicine is a historical tradition that has, for centuries, defined the very way we think about health and understand the role of the physician. Its reactive logic, even effective in crisis contexts, has left deep imprints on the doctor-patient relationship and on the limited understanding of what it truly means to be healthy.

The establishment of emergency as the core of medical practice was not accidental. The historical legacy of major epidemics and human vulnerability to unpredictable diseases created the ideal ground for medicine to adopt, almost by inertia, a model centered on urgent intervention. Epidemics like cholera, smallpox, and the devastating Spanish flu were driving forces behind the institutionalization of a medicine geared toward immediate combat, far more than toward promoting sustainable health or active prevention.

A decisive moment in this trajectory occurred in the 19th century, when hospitals began to be recognized as legitimate centers for responding to health crises. Before this, they were viewed with suspicion, associated with death, not cure. The turning point happened with the consolidation of the microbiological theories of Louis Pasteur and Robert Koch, which redefined medicine by identifying germs as disease-causing agents.

The discovery of these pathogens boosted hygiene practices and strengthened medicine as an essentially reactive and corrective activity. The logic was: if we know the enemy, we can eliminate it. It was the birth of the medical war against invisible threats, and the emergency room became the new battlefield. Medicine collected its first major scientific victories with the control of epidemics and the drop in infectious mortality, further cementing its role as a response to threat.

These victories, while signifying immense progress, generated a side effect: the disproportionate valorization of urgent intervention and the disregard for preventive and integrative approaches. Historian Charles Rosenberg, in *The Care of Strangers* (1987), describes how the hospital became the ultimate symbol of this reactive mindset—responding to the acute, the dramatic—relegating prevention to a secondary role.

Another decisive historical landmark reinforcing this emergency logic occurred during the First and Second World Wars, periods when war medicine defined new standards of clinical efficiency and powerfully reinforced the emergency mindset. Surgical techniques that save millions of lives today originated on battlefields, where the priority was not long-term health, but immediate survival. Analgesic and anesthetic medications, blood transfusions, and rapid sterilization methods are all clear examples of how military medicine consolidated the reactive paradigm in global clinical practice.

Researchers like Roger Cooter, in the publication *Medicine and Modern Warfare* (1999), demonstrate that this military heritage still deeply shapes contemporary medical education. Professional training prioritizes scenarios of maximum tension, rapid interventions, and real-time reactions, solidifying a medical culture that measures success by efficacy in the face of imminent collapse.

Even in peacetime, the medical culture continued to absorb this emergency logic without major questioning. In the post-war era, with the rise of the US and European biomedical model, hospital emergency services became the most visible face of medicine for the general public. TV series, films, and books popularized and romanticized the image of the heroic doctor always acting under extreme pressure, saving lives at the last second, with a fixed idea that medicine and emergency are almost synonymous.

This heroism of the urgent had profound effects on the medical professional identity. Many choose the profession drawn by the adrenaline and prestige it offers. This bias reinforces a cultural resistance to slower, preventive, and relational models precisely because they do not offer the same reward.

In this scenario, preventive or integrative medicine tends to be perceived as secondary. Less urgent, less exciting, and less valued. Even with public policies attempting to reverse this with primary care and educational campaigns, they face the weight of a historical tradition that glorifies rapid reaction and marginalizes the effective construction of health.

The economic cost of this tradition is well-documented. WHO reports show that hospital-centric systems consume a disproportionate fraction of healthcare resources, while community-based actions, prevention, and promotion remain chronically underfunded. The irony is, in a way, tragic: emergency medicine ultimately creates populations that are more fragile and dependent on the emergency room.

Eric Topol, in *Deep Medicine* (2019), denounces this cycle. According to him, the historically consolidated reactive medicine is ineffective against contemporary challenges like chronic diseases, which demand not urgency, but continuity, listening, and personalization. Topol warns that if medicine does not overcome this heritage, health systems are heading for collapse. This critique is shared by organizations like the OECD (Organization for Economic Co-operation and Development), which advocates for an urgent migration toward more sustainable models: preventive, integrative, and health-centered.

The COVID-19 pandemic exposed this limit. Even with the rapid response in vaccine production, the reactive logic proved flawed in preventing the crisis. Systems overloaded by decades of preventive neglect collapsed under a demand that required precisely what was never prioritized: anticipation.

Recognizing this heritage is indispensable. The history of emergency medicine is a live warning about the risks of continuing to operate within a model that saves in chaos but fails to build health. And it is this critical and urgent transition that must be made with lucidity, courage, and depth. We are here for this.

THEMATIC FOCUS: 10 PROMISES THAT SOUND GOOD BUT FAIL IN CARE

✦ **"Your tests are normal, so everything is fine."**

Why it's insufficient: Reference ranges are population statistics, not functional guarantees. People with "normal tests" may still be at high risk.

✦ **"Symptoms must be eliminated as quickly as possible."**

Why it's insufficient: Symptoms are adaptive bodily responses, often signaling regulatory processes. Eliminating them without listening can be counterproductive.

✦ **"More tests mean more safety."**

Why it's insufficient: Excessive testing increases the risk of false positives, unnecessary treatments, and clinical anxiety.

✦ **"Chronic diseases are inevitable with age."**

Why it's insufficient: Many so-called "natural" diseases are highly preventable with integrated approaches starting early.

✦ **"Medication is always the most effective treatment."**

Why it's insufficient: For a range of mild or moderate conditions, behavioral and psychosocial interventions have equal or superior efficacy, without side effects.

✦ **"Medical science is neutral and evidence-based."**

Why it's insufficient: Public policies, private funding, industry interests, and cultural biases shape what is researched, disseminated, and applied.

✦ **"The more specialization, the better the care."**

Why it's insufficient: Fragmentation among specialists without an integrative vision increases diagnostic errors and therapeutic insecurity.

✦ **"Modern medicine takes care of health."**

Why it's insufficient: The system's structure is oriented toward responding to disease, not sustaining health. Health promotion remains marginalized.

✦ **"Technology guarantees more precise diagnoses."**

Why it's insufficient: Without contextual interpretation, technology generates noise. Isolated data does not equate to clinical intelligence.

FROM THE 20TH CENTURY TO THE CULT OF INTERVENTION

The 20th century elevated this logic to a new level, with increasingly invasive procedures and intensive use of sophisticated technologies. Medicine ceased to be a response to diseases and began to incorporate an almost obsessive pursuit of control over life. Curiously, this advancement ultimately distanced medicine from the very essence of life, keeping it trapped in a constant and almost exclusive battle against death.

The discovery of antibiotics, especially penicillin by Alexander Fleming in 1928 and its popularization during World War II, symbolically marked the beginning of this new era of technological and interventional medicine. For the first time, doctors had tools capable of defeating previously fatal bacterial infections. This was the first indication that medicine could wield concrete power over death, which raised the profession's prestige and solidified the logic of intervention as a symbol of success.

The sense of triumph over nature, so characteristic of modern Western science, fueled a technological race that shaped the following decades. In the second half of the 20th century, hospitals began to resemble high-complexity laboratories, but were increasingly distant from humanized care. CT scanners, MRIs, mechanical ventilators, and hemodialysis machines became the icons of modern medicine, reinforcing the paradigm that clinical success depends on technology, not on listening, connection, or integrality.

Modern medicine sidelined the patient's experience, replacing it with the clinical objectivity of technical observation, which created a new form of medical power: a power exercised by technology that reduces the human being to the condition of an observable, measurable, and correctable body.

Physicians trained throughout the 20th century began to primarily rely on devices and procedures—far more than on clinical listening or interpersonal relationships. Medical sociologist Renée Fox, in *Experiment Perilous* (1998), shows how this excessive reliance on technique generated an institutionalized emotional distancing: doctors feel safer interacting with tool-based protocols and test results than with people.

And the rise of the modern pharmaceutical industry in the post-war decades exacerbated this process. Corticosteroids, powerful analgesics, antidepressants, and other effective drugs ushered in the era of generalized medicalization, where almost every discomfort began to have a pharmacological solution. Sociologist Peter Conrad, in *The Medicalization of Society* (2007), warns of the risks of this logic: social, emotional, and existential problems are treated as clinical disorders that demand rapid solutions. An evident example is the expansion of anxiolytic and antidepressant use. Initially viewed as revolutionary, these medications accelerated the consolidation of a clinical culture based on chemical responses, instead of therapeutic dialogue, reflection, and action on root cause and self-knowledge. According to studies in *JAMA Psychiatry* (2019), over 20% of Americans use psychotropics regularly.

Cardiology, another major representative of the interventional paradigm, also illustrates this logic. Cardiac surgery and stents revolutionized the treatment of coronary disease but promoted an excessive reliance on the immediate technical fix. According to the American Heart Association (2022), recurrence rates remain high because the invasive approach, though effective in the short term, ignores the structural causes: diet, sedentary behavior, and chronic stress. And a recommendation to the patient, "You need to eat better," does not equate to including the topic in a structured or effective manner, let us be clear. This conduct is closer to a disclaiming and total transfer of responsibility to the patient: if they don't improve their diet, they were warned.

This model achieved such institutional and economic success that it became virtually unquestionable. In *Overtreated* (2007), Shannon Brownlee exposes the recurring practice of unnecessary procedures, driven by financial motivation and because the medical culture is conditioned to intervene, even when it shouldn't. The result: increased costs, increased risks, and thousands of patients exposed to aggressive interventions without clear necessity.

Another critical point of this culture is the ideal of "survival at all costs," especially in intensive care units. Modern medicine is often oriented toward artificially prolonging life without considering the patient's quality of life, wishes, or dignity. Atul Gawande, in *Being Mortal* (2014), decries this model as medicine that offers "more treatment," but rarely offers the best treatment. The patient's will disappears under the weight of the clinical machine.

For those quick to judge, it is important to emphasize: technology is not the problem. The problem is the cult, the uncritical idolatry of a model that excludes more humane, more relational, and, crucially, more effective approaches.

THE MEDICALIZATION OF EXISTENCE: WHEN LIVING BECAME SYNONYMOUS WITH NOT DYING

As we entered the final decades of the 20th century, the model of technological and interventional medicine reached a turning point, transcending the clinical and hospital space to deeply infiltrate people's daily lives. It was in this scenario that a powerful and complex phenomenon emerged: the medicalization of existence.

The term "medicalization" was coined by sociologist Ivan Illich in his classic *Medical Nemesis* (1975), where he described, pioneeringly, how social, behavioral, and emotional problems began to be redefined as illnesses and, consequently, subjected to medical intervention. This process transformed the very experience of life into something that needed to be continuously monitored and corrected by specialists, creating a generalized social dependence on rapid medical solutions.

The impact of this medicalization altered how health itself came to be understood. Instead of being viewed as an integral potency of well-being, it became linked to the absence of clinical risks or identifiable physiological deviations. British sociologist Nikolas Rose, in *The Politics of Life Itself* (2007), shows how contemporary medicine moved away from treating visible diseases to actively seeking invisible anomalies through screenings, genetic testing, and increasingly refined biometric markers.

The explosion in early prostate cancer diagnosis via the PSA test is one such case. Although initially seen as a preventive revolution, long-term studies—such as those published by the *New England Journal of Medicine* (2012)—demonstrated that excessive screening generated a large number of unnecessary treatments with serious side effects (like impotence or urinary incontinence), without significantly increasing patients' life expectancy. Thus, a medical intervention intended to improve quality of life often deteriorated it.

With the third edition of the DSM (DSM-III) in the 1980s, diagnostic criteria expanded radically, leading to an explosion of psychiatric diagnoses. Sadness, grief, shyness, worry—common human emotions—began to be medicalized. Psychiatrist Allen Frances, who was responsible for the DSM-IV, became one of the biggest critics of this expansion. In *Saving Normal* (2013), he warns that turning life into pathology promotes a culture of illness, not health.

The impact was also economic, social, and cultural. The pharmaceutical market grew exponentially. Data from IMS Health (now IQVIA) show that the global market for antidepressants and anxiolytics virtually doubled between 2000 and 2020. The side effect of this logic is dangerous: the more daily life is viewed as a clinical dysfunction, the more the individual's autonomy weakens.

As the World Health Organization (WHO) reiterated in its landmark report, *Social Determinants of Health* (2008), direct medical interventions, while essential in certain contexts, explain only a small fraction of the variation in population health. The vast majority of factors determining health lie outside the scope of clinical medicine, residing in living conditions, work, income, social relationships, and access to healthy environments.

This situation places contemporary medicine at a conceptual and ethical crossroads: should it continue treating symptoms with "technical" responses, or finally acknowledge that health is a much deeper, systemic, and relational phenomenon? Medical philosopher Rita Charon, a pioneer of narrative medicine, argues that physicians need to relearn how to listen to stories. For her, health is the result of lives with meaning, connection, and presence.

The future of medicine depends on the courage to abandon obsolete intellectual habits and recognize that living fully is not the same as not dying. And that true care begins not with exams, but with listening, presence, and understanding all that makes life worth living.

FROM SURVIVAL TO THE MEDICINE OF FULL LIVING: AN EMERGING PARADIGM

The forceful critique made by Georges Canguilhem, in *The Normal and the Pathological*, remains absolutely relevant: a medicine that limits itself to fighting death will never be sufficient to define what it means to live well. Based on a reactive and pathological model, the healthcare system has never been able to fully respond to the complexity of healthy living, much less create conditions for people to thrive physically, mentally, and emotionally. Transitioning to another paradigm therefore requires a profound redefinition of what health truly signifies.

In recent decades, new approaches have begun to break with the reductionist logic and propose broader, more integrative visions of medical practice. Functional medicine, the biopsychosocial model, and integrative medicine are examples of concrete responses to the need to go beyond symptom suppression. Functional medicine, in particular, seeks the root causes of diseases and incorporates genetic, environmental, behavioral, and emotional factors—in contrast to the biomedical model, which treats symptoms in isolation, and is more aligned with what is known about the body's functioning.

According to the Institute for Functional Medicine, founded by Dr. Jeffrey Bland in the 1990s, full health is a state of dynamic balance—an "expanded homeostasis"—in which mind, body, environment, and relationships are in harmony. This vision is strengthened by the research of Elizabeth Blackburn, Nobel laureate in Medicine, who demonstrated in *The Telomere Effect* (2017) how emotional and social factors directly impact cellular health, aging, and longevity.

In clinical practice, this new paradigm is already manifesting concretely. Public programs and institutional initiatives are adopting expanded strategies, with multidisciplinary teams composed of psychologists, nutritionists, occupational therapists, social workers, and physical educators accompanying the patient throughout their journey. In Brazil, the Psychosocial Care Network (*Rede de Atenção Psicossocial*) integrates different levels of care to offer a more humanized service centered on the needs of people with psychological distress and harmful substance use.

And the impact of these approaches is already measurable. Reports from the American Psychological Association indicate that patients treated with biopsychosocial or integrative models have greater adherence to treatments, fewer hospital admissions, and higher satisfaction. Simultaneously, studies from the Cleveland Clinic—a global reference in integrative medicine—point to expressive reductions in healthcare costs, accompanied by gains in well-being and quality of life.

However, for these experiences to cease being exceptions and become the standard, it is indispensable to reconfigure the place where medical knowledge is born and disseminated: the classroom. It is impossible to speak of structural change without a profound reform in medical education. Traditional training teaches how to diagnose and intervene with technical precision, but little or nothing about health promotion, prevention, or deep listening to the patient in their life context. Innovative schools like Harvard Medical School and the Mayo Clinic College of Medicine are already incorporating subjects like "Clinical Communication," "Narrative Medicine," "Health and Society," and "Integrated Prevention" to prepare physicians with greater sensitivity, context, and systemic vision.

This pedagogical renewal also demands a profound shift in the doctor-patient relationship itself. The patient must cease to be an object of decision and become an active partner in the construction of their health. This requires time, empathetic listening, and attention to the life context of each individual—things that the traditional model was not designed to offer, nor are many of the healthcare solutions provided to health professionals today.

Many studies reinforce this need: research published in the *British Medical Journal* demonstrated that longer consultations are associated with better clinical outcomes and greater patient satisfaction. The *Journal of General Internal Medicine* also highlights that the use of empathetic listening significantly reduces the need for invasive interventions. A systematic review in *Patient Education and Counseling* showed that active patient involvement in healthcare improves treatment adherence and clinical results.

In Brazil, a study by the University of São Paulo showed that the doctor-patient relationship based on effective communication is directly linked to the improvement of health indicators in primary care units. Research in South Africa indicated that interventions focused on active listening in community clinics contributed to a reduction in hospital readmissions and better control of chronic diseases. There is no shortage of data.

We are, therefore, facing a decisive call. Medicine can and must go beyond mere biological survival, and turn toward the full cultivation of human life. This is how the professional of tomorrow will be able to rediscover their original meaning: to care, not just correct; to promote life, not just avert death. The path is complex, but profoundly necessary —and possible.

TIMELINE: EVOLUTION OF MEDICINE AS A REACTIVE MODEL

✦ **Ancient Greece (5th century BC)**

Historical Milestone: Hippocratic Oath

Medical Focus: Pain relief and containment of death

Insight: Despite Hippocrates proposing clinical observation, medicine was oriented toward preventing imminent physical collapse.

✦ **Ancient Rome (1st–3rd centuries AC)**

Historical Milestone: Galen systematizes medical knowledge based on humors

Medical Focus: Correction of visible imbalances

Insight: The emphasis was on intervention for acute signs, especially fevers and bleeding.

✦ Middle Ages (5th–15th centuries)

Historical Milestone: Hospitals as shelters for the dying

Medical Focus: Mitigation of death, not promotion of health

Insight: The word "hospital" comes from hospitium: shelter. Doctors also acted as spiritual figures.

✦ Renaissance (15th–16th centuries)

Historical Milestone: Vesalius inaugurates modern anatomical dissection

Medical Focus: Knowing the dead body to treat the living

Insight: Medicine advanced over cadavers. Life was understood based on the anatomy of death.

✦ 17th Century

Historical Milestone: Descartes proposes the separation of mind and body

Medical Focus: The body as a fixable machine

Insight: The mechanistic paradigm emerges: diseases as component failures.

✦ 19th Century

Historical Milestone: Pasteur and Koch found microbiology

Medical Focus: Elimination of the aggressive agent (germs)

Insight: Medicine arms itself against "invisible enemies." Focus on infection and sudden death.

. . .

✦ World Wars (1914–1945)

Historical Milestone: Consolidation of war medicine

Medical Focus: Immediate survival, field surgery

Insight: ICUs and emergency protocols derive from the military logic of saving under extreme pressure.

✦ Post-War / 1950s–70s

Historical Milestone: Explosion of the pharmaceutical industry

Medical Focus: Rapid suppression of symptoms

Insight: Anxiolytics, antibiotics, and analgesics inaugurate the era of "fixing without understanding."

✦ 1980s

Historical Milestone: Popularization of check-ups and evidence-based medicine

Medical Focus: Early detection and statistical elimination of risk

Insight: Medicine begins to measure before feeling—but still ignores life contexts.

✦ Turn of the 21st Century

Historical Milestone: Emergency of technological and interventional medicine

Medical Focus: Prolonging life at any cost

Insight: Ventilators, transplants, dialysis, stents—life extension with a fragmented vision.

✦ Present Day (2020–2025)

Historical Milestone: Crisis of meaning in the medical profession; burnout and over-medicalization; rise of AI

Medical Focus: Attempt at integration and reconnection

Insight: WHO, Harvard, Cleveland Clinic, and other institutions recognize the limits of the exclusively reactive model.

CHAPTER 3
THE COST OF MECHANISTIC REASONING

The clinical cost of the fragmented approach is not easy to measure. Protocols based on specialization work like train tracks: once a journey begins in a certain direction, any symptom that does not fit the criteria of that specific segment tends to be discarded or ignored. Medical reasoning, rather than being guided by the systemic intelligence of human complexity, begins to follow checklists of isolated symptoms —valid for simpler problems, but insufficient here. The patterns between systems—precisely those that reveal deep imbalances—remain invisible. A patient presenting with gastrointestinal, dermatological, and cognitive symptoms simultaneously will hardly be recognized as someone with a systemic inflammatory syndrome. In practice, they will most likely be referred to three distinct specialists, each confined to their silo. We must state this plainly: this prolongs suffering and diminishes the efficacy of both diagnosis and treatment.

The more specialized the care, the more myopic the assistance becomes. The healthcare system was designed to reward specialization and, in a way, punish attempts at integration. General practitioners, clinicians, and integrators are underpaid, undervalued, and frequently viewed as "less technical" than super-specialists.

A study published in the *Journal of General Internal Medicine* (2019) revealed that approximately 12 million people per year in the

US are victims of preventable diagnostic errors, and that fragmentation among specialists is one of the leading factors involved. The study shows that when a patient is seen by three or more distinct specialties, the chance of diagnostic error or omission practically doubles. What happens is that no one is responsible for the whole, and this simple fact places the patient in a vulnerable position and the service provider (whomever they may be) in a comfortable yet inefficient one.

This absence of an integrated clinical vision manifests in what are called coordination-related adverse events—harm caused not by technical error, but by the disarticulation between various specialists. The situation is this: everyone is doing their best, doing what they learned to do, and can fully defend themselves against any accusation because they did exactly what was expected and protocolized.

This logic imposes limits on the physician's own reasoning. Trained in compartments, the professional learns early on to discard variables "external" to their specialty. A cardiologist may master the electrocardiogram but does not feel authorized to consider the anxiety accelerating the heart. Specialization, which should be a virtuous deepening of knowledge, transforms into a minefield where thinking integratively is discouraged and sometimes even delegitimized.

Even more grave is the fact that this clinical fragmentation dissolves accountability for complex outcomes. When something goes wrong in the treatment of a patient with multiple symptoms and no clear diagnosis, it is common to hear the phrase "that's not my specialty." The patient is then left orphaned, without a responsible guardian for their care. No professional is trained to assume the whole, and the whole, for that very reason, is lost.

Systemic chronic diseases make this failure visible. People with lupus, fibromyalgia, metabolic syndrome, autoimmune, or neurodegenerative diseases endure a clinical ordeal. They are seen by countless specialists, receive contradictory diagnoses, and are often blamed for their lack of improvement. What is sick in this scenario is not just the body, but the model attempting to treat it.

Fragmentation also affects the doctor-patient bond itself. When every consultation is an island, little room remains to build trust or understand the deeper meanings of the illness. The patient does not feel that someone is accompanying their journey; they feel they are being "assessed," "monitored," and "referred," but not cared for.

For patients with "atypical" clinical expressions (those that do not fit the manuals), this fragmentation can be devastating. These are the ones who fall ill "off the curve," with symptoms that challenge usual classifications. And it is exactly in these cases that systemic listening is most necessary. Even in contexts where specialization is absolutely indispensable, the lack of integration compromises post-operative care, rehabilitation, adherence, and long-term care. Integration contextualizes specialty, and that too is a technique. We might say it is also a specialty: that of integrating and connecting vectors. The point is that this specialty does not yet exist, and with the spread of artificial intelligence, the Internet of Things, sensor-generated data, new exams seeing new biomarkers, advanced genetic tests, and the great revolution we are about to witness, it will be indispensable.

We are accustomed to thinking in opposites: "either this or that." But, especially here, we must break with this binary mindset. The answer often lies in the well-architected combination of different views. And this requires a willingness to listen to the other, and an architecture designed for this purpose. We will get there.

WHEN PROTOCOL OVERRIDES CLINICAL INTELLIGENCE

The technical progress of medicine in recent decades is undeniable—we have developed precise clinical protocols, sophisticated biomarkers, and diagnostic decision algorithms that surpass much of human judgment in speed and accuracy. But this precision, when disconnected from a systemic view and relational clinical intelligence, becomes a mirage. Medicine based exclusively on algorithms and compartmentalized decisions generates a false sense of control and masks the complexity of the human body and its modes of illness.

Many professionals today are trained more as "guideline enforcers" than as thinking clinicians. A study published in the *Journal of Evaluation in Clinical Practice* (Greenhalgh et al., 2014) warns of a growing substitution of clinical reasoning with the automatic compliance of guidelines. The risk is clear: the protocol becomes an end in itself, rather than an instrument adaptable to the singularity of each case. This is visible to anyone who has had to accompany a sick relative in a hospital and observe the environment's dynamics. Medical practice, in this scenario, begins to operate on an assembly line with almost robotic checkpoints. The impact of this is devastating when symptoms do not obey the rigid categories of the manuals. And with the multiplication of artificial intelligence automating tasks, the risk is automating the ineffective—merely accelerating the fragmented diagnosis.

Furthermore, with the proliferation of medical schools in recent years—many of which lack adequate spaces or hospitals for practical learning and experience—this factor gains epidemic and more worrying nuances. Future professionals risk being trained not with more understanding of the whole and of complex bodily dynamics, but with less.

A classic case: a patient arrives at the emergency room with intense fatigue, insomnia, weight loss, and diffuse muscle pain. Through triage, they see a clinician who rules out infectious causes; they are referred to a rheumatologist, who finds no criteria for fibromyalgia; they proceed to a psychiatrist, who prescribes an antidepressant, while the endocrinologist notes that the tests are "normal." The patient leaves with four stamps, a label, and no integrated understanding. And, crucially, they remain sick.

This phenomenon is the syndrome of fragmented normality—a set of "normal" findings in each isolated organ that fails to explain the patient's general problem. The term was coined in recent integrative medicine articles and illustrates the illusion generated by an exclusive focus on decontextualized data.

It is important to understand that this syndrome also persists for financial reasons: fee-for-service payment systems, still predominant even in countries with public health systems, incentivize fragmentation. The more technical steps and specialties involved, the more the system pays. Thinking of the body as a living system, with manifestations emerging from the interaction between organs, mind, and environment, becomes counterintuitive and economically disincentivized. A study conducted by the Mayo Clinic (Tai-Seale et al., 2017) revealed that, on average, doctors interrupt patients after 11 seconds of free speech. In such an environment, the idea of the physician as an integrator of information, and not just a validator of signals, is suffocated from the start of their career.

A true clinical situation helps illustrate this. A 52-year-old man with a history of mild hypertension began to present frequent headaches, inexplicable tiredness, and sporadic episodes of tingling. He was seen by cardiologists, neurologists, and endocrinologists. All tests were "normal." After four months, and thanks to the insistence of a geriatrician who still valued expanded listening, a diagnosis of chronic mercury intoxication was reached, caused by a contaminated imported supplement.

The fallacy of isolated precision also impacts the mental health of the professionals themselves. When clinical judgment is suppressed, what remains is the frustration of witnessing the patient's suffering without having a place for it in the protocols. Many doctors report feeling like mere health bureaucrats typing codes, pushing buttons. This helps explain the high rates of burnout: according to the American Medical Association (2022), more than 60% of physicians report emotional exhaustion associated with work. In Brazil, a study by the São Paulo Medical Association (2021) points out that about 57% of doctors in São Paulo present symptoms of burnout—attributed, in large part, to protocol rigidity and the absence of autonomy for personalized clinical decisions.

Complex Adaptive Systems Theory (Holland, 1995) offers an alternative lens. In it, emergent properties reside in the relationships between the parts. Applied to the clinic, this idea transforms everything: the most relevant symptom is not always in the most affected organ, but in the pattern of interaction between subsystems. The patient is not a lung with asthma, a stomach with gastritis, or a mind with anxiety. They are a dynamic field where these dimensions interact.

THEMATIC FOCUS: 7 SILENT SYMPTOMS OF CLINICAL FRAGMENTATION

✦ All tests normal, patient exhausted

- **What it seems like:** Relief: "Everything is fine."
- **What it really reveals:** Blindness to systemic syndromes,

chronic inflammatory states, and functional imbalances that do not appear in compartmentalized exams.

✦ Symptoms that "don't fit"

- **What it seems like:** Doubt about the patient: "It must be psychological."
- **What it really reveals:** The system's inability to recognize transversal manifestations and complex patterns between specialties.

✦ Constant switching of specialists without a confirmed diagnosis

- **What it seems like:** Medical diligence.
- **What it really reveals:** Collective disclaimer of responsibility: each professional treats a part, and no one cares for the whole.

✦ Prescription based solely on conduct algorithms

- **What it seems like:** Guideline-based evidence.
- **What it really reveals:** Absence of contextualized clinical reasoning. The protocol becomes a sentence, not a guide.

✦ Apps and platforms that monitor only one organ

- **What it seems like:** Technological innovation.
- **What it really reveals:** Digitization of fragmentation: technology replicating the reductionist logic of the traditional system.

✦ Medical frustration without clear explanation

- **What it seems like:** Professional stress.
- **What it really reveals:** Ethical suffering from being unable to help patients who "do not fit the protocol."

✦ Charts with excess data and absence of narratives

- **What it seems like:** Richness of information.
- **What it really reveals:** Loss of the patient's biography: decontextualized data that informs much but understands little.

THE PATIENT AS HOSTAGE OF A DISCONNECTED SYSTEM

This is the point where mechanical fragmentation becomes cruelest: when it ceases to be a limitation defined by clinical reasoning and transforms into direct suffering for those seeking care.

It is common to hear patients report that, when seeking help for diffuse pain, constant fatigue, or discomforts that "no one can explain," they are referred from one specialist to another in a kind of aimless pilgrimage. The rheumatologist looks at the blood. The orthopedist, the knee. The endocrinologist, the hormones. The psychiatrist, the symptoms. And in the end, no one looks at the patient. The multiplicity of opinions does not add up to a richer truth—it dissipates. The patient feels abandoned, not by a lack of attention, but by an excess of its segmentation.

This experience corrodes the bond, which should be the foundation of any therapeutic process. The patient feels they are being heard as a set of disconnected clinical signs. When they tell their story, they are interrupted. When they try to articulate symptoms, they are cut off by objective questions. When they mention emotions or life context, they are redirected to the exam agenda. Care becomes a "technical" inquisition.

The way we speak about the body in daily clinical practice clearly reveals the paradigm that sustains it. "Bad knee," "broken spine," "messy blood pressure," "pancreas that doesn't work"—expressions apparently harmless, but which reinforce the idea that we are the sum of parts, and that a defective part can be treated like an industrial component. The problem is that this conditions the patient to perceive themselves this way too: a machine with defects. This type of language has profound effects. The patient internalizes the diagnosis as identity ("I am hypertensive," "I am depressive," "I am diabetic"), not as someone in a process, but as someone fixed in a label. This limits their capacity for self-care, their margin for transformation, and their agency. Language shapes the experience of self.

This fragmentation extends to how we use technology. Health monitoring apps, for example, frequently reproduce this compartmentalized logic: one app for blood pressure, another for glucose, another for sleep, another for steps. Instead of promoting integration, technology reinforces the siloed view. The patient is left with the impossible task of stitching this data together and understanding how it connects. They have neither the tools, nor the time, nor the guidance. The promise of autonomy becomes a burden.

It is important to make clear that these errors are not exceptions, but symptoms of a system designed to function this way. Electronic health records are not integrated, data does not converse, specialties are isolated by walls. And protocols, instead of opening possibilities, narrow listening. The result many live with at the end of this uncomfortable equation is care that becomes a sum of bureaucratic acts.

The patient's experience is also traversed by a subtle but profound sensation: that "no one is really in charge." When a symptom worsens, they do not know who to turn to. When a test comes back altered, the specialist says: "that is for another doctor." Fragmentation generates a responsibility vacuum. And this destroys clinical safety, whether we like it or not. The problem arises when specialization becomes isolation, when deep knowledge about a part prevents recognition of the whole. It is the magnifying glass syndrome: the more one focuses on a detail, the less one sees the ensemble. And one believes that this detail *is* the whole.

This zoom-out to the true whole, however, requires more than good will; it requires structure. The current system offers no time, support, or incentives for systemic care. Therefore, this work proposes not only innovation through technology but innovation in the mindset and value proposition of healthcare services, with a reconfiguration of the foundations sustaining an ecosystem that is collapsing. And it is the numbers, research, and studies that say this. Not that it isn't a clearly observable phenomenon, but to grasp the seriousness and severity of the issue, we bring numerous evidences from various parts of the world that make this clear.

THE MYOPIA OF DISCONNECTED DATA: WHEN INFORMATION BECOMES NOISE

Exams, panels, biomarkers, and algorithms today deliver an avalanche of clinical numbers, but there has been little evolution in the capacity to make sense of this data in an integrated way. It is not about an absence of information, but its disorganization and the isolation between parts that should be conversing. Each piece of the body gets a detailed report, yet the patient remains misunderstood.

Each specialty generates its own block of data: cardiology with its ECGs and troponins, endocrinology with the hormonal cascade, pulmonology with respiratory function scores. Healthcare, with all its technical brilliance, is drowning in data that does not converse and does not generate intelligence, and is notably further behind than several other sectors.

This phenomenon was described by Van der Lei (1991), back in the early days of clinical computerization, as "data-rich but information-poor"—when there is an abundance of data, but little clinical sense. More than thirty years later, the warning remains valid. What has changed is the scale. If the excess previously came from exams, today it is amplified by predictive algorithms, wearables, monitoring platforms, and artificial intelligences operating without context. Without a meta-intelligence to integrate data into a systemic reading, the risk is that they oscillate between debris and noise.

Imagine a patient with non-specific pain, chronic tiredness, irregular sleep, but with laboratory tests all "within range." In many clinical contexts, this patient is dismissed as someone "without objective disease." But more integrated analyses—such as those done by functional medicine teams or systemic approaches—show inter-relational patterns between the HPA axis (hypothalamus-pituitary-adrenal), silent inflammation, and microbiota, which are invisible in the isolated reading of data. The failure, therefore, is not in the data, but in what one decides to see and in the absence of an integrated reading between them.

Although algorithms detect patterns with statistical precision, they often fail when exposed to complexity, where variables interact in a non-linear manner. Without a model that integrates physiology, context, and experience, data ceases to generate knowledge and produces an illusion of precision, limiting the true potential of technology. Imagine a patient with type 2 diabetes, hypertension, and mild anxiety disorder. Each specialty prescribes its intervention: one medication for glycemic control, another for blood pressure, a third for mood. Data on adherence, adverse effects, and treatment response are collected in different systems, by professionals who do not talk to each other.

This silo logic inevitably creates care gaps. The use of a beta-blocker can alter heart rate variability and be interpreted as improvement by a wearable without the pharmacological context being considered. Or: a slight increase in morning cortisol might be ignored in endocrinology, but indicative of chronic stress in psychiatry if there were a bridge between the knowledges. This contextual blindness is one of the most lethal faces of fragmented clinical reasoning.

Evidence-based medicine, while revolutionary, ended up being colonized by the same fragmentation. Many clinical trials exclude patients with comorbidities, producing evidence that only holds true in theoretical bodies. When these protocols are applied to real bodies, applicability crumbles. Isolated evidence does not hold up when applied to an interdependent system. How many doctors ask about emotional history, traumatic events, sleep patterns, work environments, affective bonds? How many hospital management software programs have fields for this? Essential information is not quantifiable, but it structures the meaning of everything that is quantified.

A survey by the Institute for Healthcare Improvement (2021) pointed out that more than 60% of serious clinical errors occur due to communication failures between areas. The collapse of clinical reading comes not from a lack of knowledge, but from a lack of cohesion between knowledges. The human body does not suffer by sectors; it suffers in a network. The analysis of integrated medical record systems shows that tools do not help this process. In a study done by the Mayo Clinic Center for Innovation, it was observed that physicians spend up to 49% of their attendance time searching for and filling in data dispersed across multiple screens and tabs. There is no "view of the patient as a system"—there is a chaotic clinical mosaic that depends on the professional's cognitive effort to assemble the puzzle.

The fragmentation of data and clinical reading needs, then, to be treated as a problem of structural architecture. Modern clinical practice needs to approach complexity sciences, which understand living systems not as fixed structures, but as adaptive networks responding to multiple stimuli, in constant interaction with the environment. In this sense, the physician ceases to be a "repairer of localized damage" to become a reader of patterns, someone capable of seeing the body as a field of forces in motion. Artificial intelligence is here to help us build this bridge, but we need to step back two paces if we want to build health-care solutions that have relevant impact at scale.

This change requires a new type of literacy: systemic clinical literacy. Training the eye to detect anomalies and recognize relationships. The challenge is no longer just diagnosing the kidney, the liver, or the thyroid—it is understanding how a patient's emotional suffering, combined with precarious sleep and an inflammatory diet, composes a picture of chronic pain that no exam captures.

THEMATIC FOCUS: 7 KEY QUESTIONS TO EVALUATE IF YOUR CLINICAL PRACTICE OR TECHNOLOGY TRULY LISTENS

✦ 1. Can the patient tell their story in their own words before being interrupted?

- Why this matters: Spontaneous narrative reveals patterns that do not appear in closed questions.
- How to evaluate: Average time to interruption (benchmark: ideal >30s), presence of open fields, freedom in the interface.

✦ 2. Does your solution collect context or just events?

- Why this matters: Decontextualized data leads to shallow clinical interpretations.
- How to evaluate: Analysis of medical record structure, capacity to store trajectory and not just symptoms.

✦ 3. Is the listening of subjectivity systematized or improvised?

- Why this matters: Subjectivity is complex data, not noise. It needs structure and method to be valued.
- How to evaluate: Presence of structured active listening protocols, trained clinical empathy, narrative anamnesis frameworks.

✦ 4. Is there recording and analysis of the patient's emotional language?

- Why this matters: Feelings shape symptoms and adherence. Ignoring emotional language is a clinical error.
- How to evaluate: Use of NLP (Natural Language Processing), voice biomarkers, or space for emotional reports in the medical record.

✦ 5. Does the technology offer integrative insights or just lists of symptoms?

- Why this matters: Clinical intelligence lies in the relationships between data, not the sum of data.
- How to evaluate: Capacity of AI or dashboard to correlate narrative patterns with physiology.

✦ 6. Does the interface accommodate nuance or impose rigidity?

- Why this matters: Systems structured simplistically force inefficient reductions.
- How to evaluate: Evaluation of "user experience" (UX) and accessibility during the patient journey in interfaces, for natural language, smart text boxes, recommendations based on behavior and available information.

✦ 7. Does the patient feel they were heard?

- Why this matters: The patient's experience is as important as the objective data.
- How to evaluate: Application of post-consultation questionnaires, listening NPS, qualitative analysis of patient feedback.

THESE QUESTIONS CAN BE USED IN DIGITAL SYSTEM REVIEW WORKSHOPS, HEALTH SERVICE DESIGN MEETINGS, OR VALIDATION PROCESSES FOR PATIENT-CENTERED HEALTHTECHS.

THE WHISPER OF THE BODY AS PRE-LABORATORY CLINICAL INTELLIGENCE

Today, a simple blood test can reveal dozens of biochemical parameters in a matter of hours. A full-body MRI can be done in a few minutes, and artificial intelligence algorithms already identify hidden patterns in images with surprising accuracy (improving every day). But this precision, however valuable, brought with it a little-debated side effect: the downgrading of clinical listening as a primary diagnostic tool. In the name of objectivity, many physicians learned to mistrust the symptom that does not appear in the report, as if the body only spoke through super-specific exams.

The patient arrives with discomfort, persistent fatigue, a bodily sensation that "something isn't right." The body whispers, but the system demands it scream to be heard. And this represents a dangerous rupture with the clinical tradition that always valued sight, touch, time, and listening as diagnostic instruments of extremely high precision.

The very concept of "pre-disease" is frequently rejected by professionals who consider only measurable and clinically established alterations as legitimate. But literature on functional medicine, lifestyle medicine, and even psychosomatics has shown that there is a relevant interval—physiologically and therapeutically—between the state of optimal health and the confirmed diagnosis. It is in this interval that many pathological processes begin to install themselves, without yet altering classic laboratory markers, and where early interventions can change the course of clinical history. So, the more patients demand a more effective vision, the more professionals will need to move to generate value for the patient.

Detailed anamnesis (history taking), when well conducted, remains one of the most powerful tools in medicine—and today is often only available to those who can pay dearly for a professional and differentiated treatment. A study by the University of São Paulo (USP) in 2020 demonstrated that 78% of diagnoses can be made based on a good clinical history, highlighting the importance of this practice in the Brazilian health context. More recent studies confirm this: research published in the *African Journal of Primary Health Care & Family Medicine* in 2023 revealed that 82% of diagnoses in primary care settings were correct based on a thorough anamnesis, even before complementary exams were performed. Another study, from 2024, released in the *Asia Pacific Journal of Public Health*, demonstrated that physicians applying advanced active listening techniques and integrative clinical reasoning increased diagnostic accuracy in complex cases.

It is frequent that women with symptoms such as loss of libido, inexplicable weight gain, menstrual irregularities, and mood changes have these attributed to emotional factors or expected aging, when in fact they may be related to subtle imbalances of estrogen, progesterone, or thyroid not detectable by traditional metrics. Functional endocrinology has already developed various models to understand these conditions, but still encounters resistance in conventional clinical contexts.

Even in more acute contexts, pre-laboratory listening makes a difference. Patients with acute myocardial infarction may report "atypical" symptoms days before the event (mild arm pain, unusual fatigue, sudden anxiety) that only become intelligible after the severe outcome. The body signals, but the clinical eye needs to be trained to decipher these signs.

In Chinese medicine, the pulse, tongue, skin coloration, and brightness of the eyes have always been considered legitimate clinical markers. And even if many of these criteria do not have a direct translation in laboratory exams, they cannot be discarded as pseudoscience. Research in physiology and neuroscience has rediscovered validity in these signals as indicators of the organism's autonomic, inflammatory, and neuroendocrine state. The synergy between ancestral medicine and contemporary science, when done with criteria, is a sophistication of care.

It is necessary to rescue the sensitivity of clinical reasoning, flattened by protocols and by a declared "rush" that serves as an answer to avoid looking at opportunities and crises. New technologies can be allies if designed to amplify listening, and promising models already exist: the Ellipsis Health project in the US developed algorithms detecting early signs of mental distress based on natural speech analysis in remote consultations. The system transcribes and interprets pauses, hesitations, intonations, and emotional vocabulary. It has already been tested in primary care clinics and showed accuracy superior to 80% in screening mild depressions that would go unnoticed by traditional scales.

Taliaz, an Israeli healthtech, crosses genetic data, self-reported patterns, and digital clinical history to propose personalized mental health treatments. Instead of trial and error, very common in antidepressant prescription, the algorithm suggests interventions adjusted to individual physiology. The laboratory exam is present, but contextualized.

In Brazil, a group of doctors from the Santa Casa de Misericórdia in São Paulo developed algorithms capable of identifying, through a short sample of the patient's voice (a few seconds are sufficient for good accuracy), signs of depression and anxiety. The solution is nascent, and in personal conversation with one of the creators, it became clear how seriously the accuracy and potential of the models are taken; a detailed article published in *Scire Salutis* shows promising results in detail.

In Germany, Ada Health is being used by patients as a symptom self-assessment tool supported by AI. When used in supervised clinical contexts, it proved useful in the early identification of ambiguous patterns meriting clinical attention. By giving language to discomforts even before they become diagnoses, platforms like this become allies in the field of functional detection, which is, by essence, pre-laboratory.

These projects reveal that pre-laboratory clinical listening is a vector of innovation. And it must be potentiated by emerging technologies. Tools like heart rate variability (HRV) biosensors, continuous glucose monitors, and symptom tracking apps are already being used by clinicians to detect dysfunction patterns, silent inflammation, and circadian rhythm alterations, all clinical predictors preceding laboratory alterations. More than identifying anomalies, this new clinical model proposes tracking physiological coherence.

But this listening requires a revolution in the concept of clinical data. Signs like fragmented sleep, tiredness upon waking, appetite variation, night sweats, inexplicable irritability, or mood fluctuations are relevant; they are code. Code of a body that has not yet collapsed, but is no longer in equilibrium. And regenerative clinical practice begins exactly there: in the blind spot of traditional practice.

REBUILDING THE SYSTEMIC VIEW OF CARE

The good news is that, despite the critical picture, the transformation has already begun. Hospitals, startups, research centers, and some medical curricula are beginning to redesign the view of the body and of care. The mechanistic view, though still hegemonic, already encounters resistance in practices seeking to reconnect clinical reasoning with the complexity of the human organism. It is no longer utopian to speak of interdisciplinary rounds based on systemic patterns—there are hospitals doing them. Nor is the idea of artificial intelligence acting as a co-pilot for real-time clinical decisions, expanding the physician's field of vision and reducing blindness caused by segmentation, fiction any longer.

An interesting case is that of the Mount Sinai Health System in New York, where researchers use predictive AI models to analyze multiple clinical signals in parallel—from laboratory tests to behavioral patterns recorded in charts—and generate alerts crossing specialties. The goal is to reveal hidden connections between seemingly unconnected symptoms. Technology, here, acts as a seamstress and reconfigures medical reasoning itself.

Stanford Medicine has implemented pilot protocols where multidisciplinary teams jointly evaluate patients with complex and persistent symptoms—especially in cases of autoimmune diseases, long COVID, or multisystemic syndromes. The focus is not to "refer," but to compose an integrated view of the patient-system. The result: more precise diagnoses, less iatrogenesis, and greater therapeutic adherence. This logic only sustains itself when the model abandons the fragmented organizational chart and acts as a coordinated clinical organism. Here, algorithms do not point to a single answer but expand clinical reasoning and help doctors build meaning.

In this scenario, we see the evolution of tools with even greater disruptive potential: clinical conversational AI. Unlike models focused on prediction or automation, this AI interacts with the doctor or patient in natural language, understanding context, crossing sources, and suggesting integrated hypotheses. Google Health tests models of this type, trained not only with biometric data but with real interactions between doctors and patients to understand how clinical reasoning forms and how it can be amplified with assistive intelligence, rather than replaced by a fixed protocol. Recently, it advanced in developing Med-PaLM, a language model specifically aimed at healthcare applications. Med-PaLM was trained on a wide variety of clinical scenarios, including electronic health record notes and real use cases, with the goal of improving the precision and relevance of answers in medical contexts. Google Health formed strategic partnerships with renowned health institutions to refine the model with direct feedback from professionals in the field, to increase information accuracy and the capacity to provide understandable and contextualized explanations for doctors and patients.

These conversational models have proven effective in constructing intelligent clinical summaries, where AI synthesizes the history of a patient with multiple comorbidities. But more than summaries, these AIs are beginning to act as facilitators of clinical empathy, suggesting broader questions, alerting to symptoms that escape the specific doctor's specialty, and even translating the patient's suffering into language accessible to the health team.

The Clinical AI Companion project, implemented in Japan in partnership with universities and medical technology companies, acts as a continuous clinical assistant, accompanying the patient on their journey through different specialties, maintaining an integrated history, detecting systemic patterns, and alerting to ruptures in clinical coherence between distinct diagnoses. The function is not to judge the professional, but to coordinate the patient's narrative in multiple aspects that a specialist alone cannot achieve.

In Brazil, initiatives like that of Pardini Tech, the digital arm of the Hermes Pardini group, are beginning to implement integrative intelligence platforms that gather laboratory data, clinical histories, and patient behavioral data into dashboards accessible by different professionals. The solution already shows a reduction in redundant exams, faster diagnoses, and higher perceived quality by patients.

Fragmentation, which was useful for building medical knowledge, has today become a dangerous limit. And the only way out is not to abandon science, but to evolve it: from a science of separation to a science of articulation. As Edgar Morin said, "it is not knowledge that we lack, but the art of organizing knowledge."

It is admirable how far we have advanced with specialization. But now, with so much accumulated knowledge, available technology, and systemic understanding of the body, we have the chance to make a leap never seen before in the history of medicine. Conversational AI can become the new clinical magnifying glass that amplifies the patient as a narrative, as a system, as a presence. It is this magnifying glass that can reveal what previously slipped through the fingers of specialization.

A body can be divided into parts to be studied, but it can only be healed when it becomes whole again.

CHAPTER 4
NEGLECTING WHAT DOESN'T SHOW UP ON TESTS

THE SYMPTOM DISCARDED BECAUSE IT DID NOT FIT THE TEST

The dominant biomedical model was consolidated upon a premise that permeates all clinical practice: that the value of data is directly associated with its capacity to be objectively measured. In other words, only that which can be recorded in an exam, scanned in an image, or reduced to a number is clinically valid. This logic is a direct inheritance from positivist medicine, which sought distance from subjectivity to approach the scientific ideal of neutrality. But this attempt to be more precise and quantifiable ended up producing the exact opposite: the elimination of lived experience as clinical data.

The patient's report, which should be the starting point for investigation, is frequently treated as noise. This not only impoverishes care but compromises its efficacy. Conditions such as fibromyalgia, endometriosis, myalgic encephalomyelitis (known as chronic fatigue syndrome), long COVID, and so many others share the same stigma: they are frequently unclassifiable in conventional exams. Consequently, the patient begins to be held responsible for their own pain.

In a seminal article published in the *Journal of Evaluation in Clinical Practice*, researcher Trisha Greenhalgh warns of the "colonization of the clinic by metrology," where medicine surrenders to a dictatorship of evidence that excludes everything that cannot be tabled. According to Greenhalgh, this limits clinical intelligence and leads to a "progressive disinvestment in listening," with direct consequences on diagnostic precision.

This erasure also exposes a veiled hierarchy of knowledges. The professional's technical knowledge is systematically placed above the patient's embodied experience. A perverse asymmetry then emerges: the patient needs to convince the doctor that they are indeed sick or that they know something relevant about themselves. It is what Annemarie Mol, in her theory of the "multiple body," calls the medicine of authority, where the feeling body is silenced by the measured body. Curiously, this same practice that scorns the subjective is capable of treating marginal biometric data with extreme rigor. A slight cholesterol increase can lead to years of statin treatment, while years of pain without apparent cause are treated with indifference. The numerical body gains precedence over the lived body. We forgot, at some point, the historical limitations of our measuring tools and decided that everything not measurable is less relevant.

The silencing of experience directly affects clinical outcomes. Studies show that patients who feel heard and understood adhere more to treatment and have better therapeutic results. What is at stake here is clinical efficacy, and healthcare that discards subjectivity is healthcare that is less precise, less responsive, and more prone to error.

In chronic diseases, this exclusion becomes even graver. As these are conditions modulated by life history, emotions, and environmental stressors (topics we will delve into further on), treating them as purely biomedical entities is a structural error. It is no coincidence that so many of them remain classified as "without defined cause" or "without cure."

More recently, researchers have been proposing the concept of an operationalized subjectivity: the effort to systematically include experience in clinical assessment models. This ranges from motivational interviews to digital data collection tools, passing through scales that contextualize pain.

Complex systems medicine points in the same direction: subjectivity is an inseparable component of physiological dynamics. A living, adaptive, and self-organized system, like the human body, cannot be understood if reports are dissociated from their manifestations.

THE EXTINCTION OF MEANINGFUL ANAMNESIS

Anamnesis (taking a medical history) has always been one of the noblest pillars of the clinical act. Listening to the patient's story with attention and time was a central gesture of medical practice, like a ritual of welcoming and validation. Today, this space has been corroded. It has transformed into a timed interrogation, dominated by closed questions, electronic protocol filling, and time control. Instead of narrative and listening, we have a checklist, a hurried data collection, and a rigid script that interrupts the patient before their story even emerges.

By breaking the patient's narrative thread, the professional loses fundamental clues—details that do not appear in exams but are in the way the story is told, in the pauses, in the silences, in the connections between seemingly disconnected events. The phenomenon of missed diagnoses has grown in recent decades, and a significant part is associated with failure in initial clinical listening (Graber, 2005; Schiff, 2009). These are diagnoses lost not due to lack of exams or technology, but due to absence of time, attention, and openness to patient complexity.

Listening is an instrument of diagnostic precision. Narrative medicine has demonstrated that patients who have space to tell their story are better understood, better treated, and more prone to adhering to treatments. It is not about "alternative medicine," but about an expanded form of clinical rationality. Listening is a valuable process of collecting complex data: subjective, contextual, symbolic in nature. When it is replaced by protocols of "standardized questions," like systems automating triage with shallow forms, the loss of clinical information is inevitable.

But diverse experiences are repositioning listening at the center of care. Structured narrative consultations, adopted in centers like Columbia University Medical Center, train doctors to hear entire stories before intervening. In another field, digital diaries integrated into medical records are emerging, allowing the patient to record their experience between consultations (feelings, events, perceptions) for the professional to incorporate this dimension. According to studies done in integrative primary care contexts, these tools are associated with higher care adherence and lower readmission rates.

In the universe of emerging technologies, the use of artificial intelligence applied to contextualized clinical listening is gaining strength. Platforms like Suki, which uses voice recognition and AI to record anamnesis conversationally, or Nuance Dragon Ambient eXperience, which automates consultation documentation based on passive and continuous listening, seek to return the freedom to listen to the doctor while the machine writes. It is still early to evaluate larger real impacts, but what is already perceived is that clinical conversational AI, when well-calibrated, can function as an "invisible secretary," returning full attention to the professional. Some technological solutions even attempt to expand listening. Kintsugi Health developed a vocal analysis system based on machine learning, capable of detecting early signs of psychological distress like depression and anxiety through subtle speech patterns. The proposal is not to replace the human ear, but to offer a complementary layer of perception, which may or may not be clinically validated, but which expands the field of attention.

In experiences like that of Beth Israel Deaconess Medical Center, patients report greater respect, stronger bonds, and greater willingness to continue treatment with the same professional. In an increasingly connected world, it is difficult to justify that the medical record is still not, by default, accessed, commented on, and adjusted by the patient themselves.

But perhaps the most sensitive point is this: anamnesis is not just about the clinical past; it is about the relational present of the consultation. When the doctor truly listens, the patient feels they matter. When interrupted, the space becomes technical, cold, and dehumanized. This affects the patient's very willingness to reveal symptoms, fears, discomforts. And once again we must bring up medical training as a vector: most medical schools teach little (or nothing) about narrative. Knowing how to listen, interpret, and integrate personal stories is not considered a central competence, although it determines the quality of clinical practice. In many schools, time dedicated to reading images exceeds that dedicated to human listening. It is not a coincidence; it is a structural choice.

Even more serious is when institutions reinforce the blockage of listening. Consultations lasting eight minutes, medical records that only accept codes, productivity goals measured in number of visits. In this environment, listening to the patient is almost an act of disobedience. The professional who attempts to listen calmly finds themselves penalized for delaying the flow, compromising the schedule, or straying from protocol. Listening has become, paradoxically, an act of disobedience, when it is precisely listening that can save us. In a world saturated with data, what is missing is meaning. And the only thing the machine does not yet fully understand is the human significance of what traverses us. Listening well is, today, a countercultural gesture—and, perhaps, the most potent one a health professional can offer.

When AI assumes the bureaucracy, space remains for the encounter. When algorithms organize data without suffocating the subject, we have more precision, not less. And when the medical record allows for nuance and narrative, it transforms into a truer clinical mirror. And when the doctor relearns to listen, they diagnose better and rebuild trust. The medicine of the future needs to listen to the past, and the past is in the voice of those who suffer.

THEMATIC FOCUS: FROM THE CLINIC THAT SILENCES TO THE CLINIC THAT LISTENS - HEALTHCARE CONTRASTS

✦ Patient Listening

- **Classic Model:** Reduced to objective complaints and clocked time.
- **Integrative Model:** Includes body language, pauses, ambivalence, narratives.

✦ Medical Record

- **Classic Model:** Record of data, codes, and objective findings.

- **Integrative Model:** Record also of perceptions, context, bonds, and history.

✦ Symptom Validation

- **Classic Model:** Only if quantifiable or visible in exams.
- **Integrative Model:** Even subjective manifestations are considered clinical.

✦ Diagnosis

- **Classic Model:** Focus on what can be named, coded, treated.
- **Integrative Model:** Focus on building shared meaning about the illness.

✦ Intervention

- **Classic Model:** Protocol-driven, guideline-based.
- **Integrative Model:** Adjustable, based on biography and life moment.

✦ Clinical Time

- **Classic Model:** Linear, productive, efficiency-oriented.
- **Integrative Model:** Circular, oriented toward listening, construction, and trust.

✦ Patient Role

- **Classic Model:** Passive object reporting symptoms.
- **Integrative Model:** Active subject interpreting, proposing, and deciding with the professional.

✦ Conception of Cure

- **Classic Model:** Disappearance of symptoms or dysfunction.
- **Integrative Model:** Recovery of meaning, functional capacity, and vitality.

THE MEDICINE THAT DOUBTS WHAT DOESN'T FIT THE EXAM

Medical records register "cases of chronic lower back pain," "patient with depressive profile," "gastrointestinal symptoms without defined cause"—each excerpt documented in isolation. Collectively, what emerges is a mosaic without stitching. The subject is fragmented linguistically and clinically, and language contributes to maintaining the split. The doctor reading the record sees a series of overlaps. The fact is that patients followed by multiple specialists have an increased risk of conflicting prescriptions. The absence of a longitudinal and integrative view of care multiplies the risk of drug interactions, divergent diagnoses, and inappropriate resource use. Fragmentation is a threat to patient safety and health systems.

Patients with chronic diseases lacking a clear biological marker face not only physical pain but clinical skepticism. The absence of coordination between doctors leads patients to abandon care plans due to cognitive and emotional saturation. When each specialist proposes contradictory paths, the patient is thrown into a labyrinth, needing to choose whom to believe, and whom to disobey. What is missing, as Professor Danielle Ofri points out in *What Patients Say, What Doctors Hear*, is an ecology of care: an organization of clinical knowledge that crosses disciplines without breaking the thread of the human narrative.

This fraying worsens when the very structure of care forces the patient to repeat the same report at every consultation. "Did I already tell you this?", "Did you see my previous exams?", "Didn't my other doctor speak to you?" are questions repeated in clinics with almost comic frequency, were they not tragic. This narrative fatigue, the sensation of having to re-explain oneself constantly, is, in itself, a type of violence.

In contrast, there are concrete experiences showing the clinical potential of integrated listening. A study conducted at the Cleveland Clinic Center for Functional Medicine compared patients with chronic diseases treated by interdisciplinary teams with patients treated by general practitioners. The results showed consistent improvements in inflammatory markers, medication adherence, and reduction in reports of emotional distress. The differentiator? Expanded consultation time, shared listening, and collaboratively built anamnesis.

Other initiatives gain traction in clinics adopting the Narrative-Based Medicine model, such as Penny Brohn UK and the Program in Narrative Medicine at Columbia University. The patient is invited to tell their story even before the first blood pressure measurement, and the body is seen in its behavioral, emotional, and systemic dimension. Technology, instead of fragmenting, is used to map relationships between symptoms, life events, and existential contexts, using visual tools, assistive AI, and narrative databases. They are not alternative; they are evolutionary. In a world where chronic diseases and multifactorial conditions are the rule, continuing to treat isolated parts is a slow—and expensive—way to fail.

THEMATIC FOCUS: THE 3 LEVELS OF LISTENING

1. Descriptive Listening — Pure Data

Capture of objective variables and raw patient report.

Characteristics: Input without interpretation, closed questions, absence of context.

Examples and applications: Apps recording pain on a 1-10 scale, heart rate, spot glucose.

2. Contextual Listening — Relational Data

Connection between data and life history. Listening considers the "why" and "with whom."

Characteristics: Interface with narrative fields, AI recognizing patterns over time, longitudinal medical record.

Examples and applications: Digital diaries, smart anamnesis with NLP, systems with symptomatic timelines.

3. Integrative Listening — Meaningful Data

Listening is used to generate complex clinical understanding and guide decision-making.

Characteristics: Active interpretation, use of generative AI for personalized synthesis, subject-centered decision support.

Examples and applications: Tools like Ada Health (with narrative + symptom interpretation), solutions with AI suggesting integrated hypotheses (Gyant, HealthOS).

> Many solutions claim to listen but are restricted to Level 1, where data is collected but not understood. The true digital revolution in health begins in the leap to Level 3—where listening becomes precision clinical technology and relational potency.

THE AESTHETICS OF INNOVATION WITHOUT CLINICAL FUNCTION

The transition from traditional medicine to digital medicine brought exponential advances in precision, reach, and efficiency. But while we gained sensors, algorithms, and platforms, we lost—or worse, neglected—the subject who falls ill. The fundamental error of many current healthtechs lies not in the technology itself, but in the premise sustaining them: they treat the patient as data, not as a subject. In the name of automation, scalability, and standardization, and still with a simplistic vision of what it means to promote health, many digital health systems simply replicate the fragmented logic of traditional biomedicine.

Health monitoring apps that have become popular in recent years offer tracking of sleep, heart rate, steps, mood, and even caloric intake—

but, in most cases, without any integration between these dimensions. The user is bombarded with graphs but rarely finds meaning. As Deborah Lupton, a theorist of digital health sociology, states, we are living a "datafication of the body" without semantics, without meaning: data is collected, but its interpretation is quite limited. The body becomes a dashboard but does not gain a contextual interpretation. The result is an illusion of self-care that is quite shallow and fragile, based on decontextualized metrics.

This logic affects not only the moment of care but the entire clinical analysis. Medical decision support systems, increasingly used, rely on massive databases, but ones generally impoverished of context. In the UK, algorithms used by the public health system for cardiovascular risk screening prioritized demographic variables and laboratory exams but did not consider factors like informal family history, chronic emotional conditions, or previous experiences of health system use—all fundamental to understanding true risk. The result was a systematic bias in preventive counseling, disproportionately harming ethnic minorities and patients with lower health literacy.

Projects like that of the company Ellipsis Health, which uses AI (NLP) to identify markers of depression and anxiety from tone and voice rhythm, show that it is possible to create systems that understand and interpret with impressive precision.

Patients who do not recognize themselves in the presented data tend to mistrust recommendations. A study published in the *Journal of the American Medical Informatics Association* (2022) showed that patients who feel their devices do not "capture the truth" about their experience report lower treatment adherence, even when physiological data is correct. What is at stake here is not the precision of numbers, but the sensation of presence and recognition. Your sleep or glucose data does not say everything about your anguish, your fear, your biography.

But there are promising paths. Startups like Wysa (India/UK), using conversational AI for empathetic listening in mental health, are redesigning digital care. These systems analyze language, emotion, and reporting patterns, generating qualitative insights as well. In the US, Cityblock Health adopts medical records allowing the patient to record what matters most in their care, even if it fits no traditional field. In

Brazil, hospitals like Sírio-Libanês initiated experiments with context-sensitive triage, including subjective aspects from the start.

The question is no longer "what can we measure?", but "what do we need to understand?". This requires a new paradigm: one that recognizes subjective data as part of clinical truth. That treats listening as technology. And that places artificial intelligence at the service of meaning—not empty automation.

THE RETURN OF LISTENING AS PRECISION TECHNOLOGY

For a long time, listening was considered an act of empathy. And it is. But it is also—and perhaps more than ever—an act of clinical precision. Listening is one of the most neglected technologies in the clinical arsenal today.

And it needs to be designed, trained, refined as a structured competence. Instead of following rigid scripts of questions, the professional learns to identify narrative archetypes, gaps, habits—clues that do not appear in exams but say much about the state of health. A patient describing pain as "being caught in a trap" or "carrying an invisible chain" may be revealing, beyond physical discomfort, a psychic experience marked by helplessness, fear, or chronic emotional withdrawal. These narrative clues help the clinician formulate more complex, more human, and more relevant hypotheses.

And this type of listening can be systematized. At Harvard, the Medical School already includes narrative medicine and active listening disciplines in the curriculum. In Toronto, pilot projects with extended consultations have shown significant reduction in unnecessary test prescriptions and increased therapeutic adherence. In Brazil, the Hospital das Clínicas has been testing a structured listening tool mediated by generative AI, where the patient reports their trajectory and the system suggests clinical summaries based on linguistic and correlational patterns.

And this is where technology can become its catalyst. New generations of conversational artificial intelligence, based on transformers and large language models (LLMs), allow information to be collected and interpreted with contextual depth. When well-designed, these tools "listen" to the patient and help the doctor listen better. They systematize what is said, point out inconsistencies, reveal previously unattainable symptomatic clues, without reducing report complexity to the rigidity of a binary form. MIT's voice biomarkers project detects depressive symptoms and signs of cognitive decline from subtle variations in the patient's voice. Kintsugi integrates AI-based emotional listening into telemedicine systems, generating alerts of hidden, unverbalized suffering.

But caution is needed. Automating listening without criteria can generate an illusion of listening. The design of these technologies must be born from a commitment to expanding the human. The doctor cannot be a passive spectator of what the AI heard. They must be the final interpreter of the patient's story, while technology paves the bond. Listening better demands better tools, but also a willing, trained, and ethically implicated ear.

More than listening, one must know what to do with what is heard. This involves training. Courses in clinical design, discourse analysis, medical anthropology, and even literature should compose the foundation of a professional dealing with people. As Trisha Greenhalgh says, "every doctor is a hermeneutician—their job is to interpret, not just measure." By transforming this skill into technical competence, we break the dichotomy between science and sensitivity. They are inseparable when we treat a body, a life.

Reintegrating the subject is also preventing errors. Not listening to symptoms straying from the expected, not considering social context, ignoring the patient's previous history: all this contributes to tragic outcomes, which could have been treated early if the patient's history had been considered.

And as digital health spreads, listening will be increasingly distributed: chatbots, apps, sensors, AI assistants, voice reports, online forms. The true challenge will be stitching these speeches into a single coherent narrative. This is where AI can operate as a curator of meaning —connecting fragments, organizing patterns, revealing absences. But this only gains potency if there is a professional prepared to deal with this narrative density.

Finally, rescuing listening requires a cultural shift. Listening well is work. It demands time, attention, presence, openness to not knowing.

And it also demands structure: workflows allowing listening, protected times for it, remuneration models valuing bond quality.

THEMATIC FOCUS: 2 PATHS FOR DIGITAL HEALTH - WHAT SEPARATES MONITORING FROM UNDERSTANDING

✦ Data

✘ Predominant Model: Monitoring of objective physiological data (heart rate, sleep, steps, glucose, etc.).
✓ Emerging Integrative Solutions: Integration of objective and subjective data based on life history, context, and patient narrative patterns.

✦ Underlying Epistemology

✘ Predominant Model: Technocratic positivism—what cannot be measured does not exist.
✓ Emerging Integrative Solutions: Complex epistemology—values singularity and narrative as clinical data.

✦ Base Technology

✘ Predominant Model: Apps and wearables focused on isolated biometrics.
✓ Emerging Integrative Solutions: Platforms with generative AI, NLP, and voice biomarkers to interpret the human report.

✦ Practical Example

✘ Predominant Model: Sleep monitoring by noise and movement, but missing insomnia from silent anxiety (Apple Health, Fitbit, Samsung Health, glucose-centric apps).
✓ Emerging Integrative Solutions: AI trained to interpret subjective diaries and correlate emotional patterns with insomnia cycles, narrative

consultations (e.g., OpenNotes), integrative NLP (e.g., Ada Health, Gyant, Kintsugi).

✦ Interface Design

✘ Predominant Model: Extreme 'formularization': multiple choice, rigid fields, absence of free narrative.
✓ Emerging Integrative Solutions: Structured open fields, natural language with semantic intelligence.

✦ Patient Role

✘ Predominant Model: Supplier of physiological data.
✓ Emerging Integrative Solutions: Co-author of clinical reasoning: their reports guide hypotheses and therapeutic strategies.

✦ Professional Role

✘ Predominant Model: Executor of protocols based on isolated or poorly connected data.
✓ Emerging Integrative Solutions: Clinical-communicational interpreter crossing objective and subjective data to generate systemic understanding.

✦ Suffering Capture

✘ Predominant Model: Extremely low—what lacks a marker is not prioritized.
✓ Emerging Integrative Solutions: High—recognizes pain, multifactorial suffering (e.g., voice analysis in mental health - MIT).

✦ Attention to Complexity

✘ Predominant Model: Reduction of patient to isolated variables.

✓ Emerging Integrative Solutions: Recognition of health as a complex and relational adaptive system.

✦ Emotional Integration

✘ Predominant Model: Non-existent—emotion ignored as clinical data.
✓ Emerging Integrative Solutions: Expanding—AI integrating mood, emotion, language metaphors.

✦ Implementation Cost

✘ Predominant Model: Initially lower, with high hidden cost due to errors and abandonment.
✓ Emerging Integrative Solutions: Demands higher initial investment, but increases adherence and care sustainability.

CHAPTER 5
DISEASE AS A BUSINESS MODEL

DISEASE AS A PRODUCT: A LOGIC DISGUISED AS CARE

The ecosystem that has formed around healthcare has transformed disease into the raw material of an expanding market. This is a fact documented in economic reports, public health studies, and journalistic investigations. Healthcare costs have skyrocketed in recent decades, even in countries with highly specialized and advanced technologies, without population well-being indicators keeping pace with this curve. This mismatch reveals a mechanism designed to keep the patient within the system.

The problem lies not only in how we treat disease but in how it has become the epicenter of the entire healthcare structure. Procedures, hospitalizations, exams, and prescriptions are today the supporting axes of hospital and pharmaceutical revenue. This does not mean that doctors or managers are driven by deliberate greed—many are victims or prisoners of this same logic. But the architecture of the current model was designed to reward spot repair. In marketing terms, the healthy patient does not generate revenue.

The fee-for-service model, predominant in much of the world, clearly exemplifies this logic. In it, the professional or institution is remunerated per procedure performed, not per result achieved. Each consultation, exam, or procedure becomes a revenue line, regardless of whether the patient actually improves. This transforms care into a fragmented and potentially inflated production chain. A study published in the *Journal of Health Economics* (2022) confirmed that clinics operating on this model perform, on average, more interventions per patient, without proportional gain in clinical outcomes. Oh, and yes, it also carries a conflict of interest: for the institution providing "health" services, the more exams the patient undergoes, the better. What protects the patient from unnecessary exams and procedures? Or from the choice of one medication over another more effective one for the case due to laboratory commissions? Individual ethics? The patient today is not only vulnerable and unprotected, but the very dynamic of this market favors and stimulates these actions.

The pharmaceutical industry operates in parallel under another logic: that of the blockbuster. Medications generating billions per year are prioritized over non-pharmacological solutions, even when the latter prove more effective in the long term. An investigation revealed that drugs for cholesterol, type 2 diabetes, and mild depression continue to be widely prescribed, despite evidence of the superiority, in various contexts, of interventions based on lifestyle, psychosocial support, or functional nutrition. Chronic disease ceases to be an adversity and becomes a stable financial asset. Here, we are not criticizing capitalism, nor would it make sense to. But what we bring is that the "health" market possesses a particularity that other markets do not: it deals directly with lives. Simple as that. This means that any decision needs, in theory, to pass through an ethical sieve as rigorous as that of laboratory exams, for example. An institution or professional proposing to work with health and making decisions that knowingly disadvantage health, or where more efficient alternatives in the patient's interest exist, needs to be widely debated, if not combated.

In Brazil, a study by Fiocruz (2021) reinforces this portrait. The survey demonstrated that although health promotion programs—such as guided physical activity or nutrition workshops—have proven impact on chronic diseases, they receive a tiny fraction of the investment directed toward medicating these same conditions. The inversion of priorities reveals a system that recognizes the clinical value of prevention but does not remunerate it. Consequently, recurrent illness is more profitable than its interruption.

The logic is brutal but transparent. In 2018, a report from a major bank sent to investors caused a scandal by stating, bluntly, that curative gene therapies could be "problematic for the business model," precisely because they eliminate the need for continuous treatments. The phrase is shocking, but it makes our point clear: what is at stake is the financial sustainability of an industry that depends on the continuity of illness to maintain its machinery and be able to remunerate its executives and partners. There is no problem in making money. There is a problem in making money from decisions that will kill, sicken, or keep people sick. And this, my dear reader, is more normalized and neglected than we realize.

The hospital, which should be the sanctuary of cure and care, is often the epicenter of this productivist and negligent logic. Length of stay, number of exams per patient, and frequency of return visits become institutional performance metrics. Reports from the Institute for Healthcare Improvement indicate that up to 30% of procedures in US hospitals are considered unnecessary or of doubtful clinical value. In a system that rewards those who do more, results inevitably take a back seat.

Natural conditions, such as passing sadness, aging, childhood restlessness, metabolic variations, or basic nutrient deficiencies, are repackaged as diagnoses with an ICD code, name, protocol, and treatment. This means questioning the transformation of every nuance of life into a pathology with a prescription, while complex pathology is not treated broadly. Psychiatrist Joanna Moncrieff denounces in her studies how selective serotonin reuptake inhibitors (SSRIs) were promoted as a panacea without solid evidence of superiority to placebos in many mild cases.

In the Brazilian context, the phenomenon repeats itself. Early and unnecessary hospitalization, hyper-inflated surgical indication, and the rarity of preventive programs in private health systems are faces of the same mechanism. The National Supplemental Health Survey (2021) showed that less than 12% of private plan users received any formal health promotion intervention in the last year. What does not generate revenue does not receive priority.

Regulation itself is captured by this logic. Sanitary agencies and public policies concentrate efforts on validating curative therapies, while integrative or social actions suffer from scarce funding, institutional distrust, and low scientific legitimacy. What counts as "science" is filtered by an evidence matrix favoring pharmacological interventions of rapid, measurable, and sellable response, rather than less immediate approaches with deeper population impact.

And even when there is evidence, the game is not neutral. John Ioannidis, in his work on scientific integrity, showed how a good part of published studies largely consumed by health professionals to define the drugs they will prescribe suffers from funding bias or methodological design oriented to favor the sponsor. The "cure," in this observed dynamic, ceases to offer integral resolution of suffering and prioritizes the maintenance of parameters within controllable ranges. Medicine approaches the industrial logic of maintenance—the most interesting for the pharmaceutical industry and also the least interesting for the patient. Wait, do we have a problem here?

Health is the organism's capacity to adapt in the face of adversity. Vitality is correlated with adaptability. By confusing normality with statistics, today's medicine transforms fully functional bodies into potential patients. The consequence is that we treat as a failure what is often just a legitimate variation of life or a sign of something larger needing investigation (often with active listening) before becoming a prescription.

The manipulation of diagnostic criteria itself is one of the subtlest and most perverse gears of this model. When thresholds defining what is "disease" are lowered without broad debate, we are artificially widening the market of patients. An emblematic example is the revision of arterial hypertension diagnostic parameters promoted by American guidelines in 2017. With the simple reduction of cut-off values for systolic and diastolic pressure, 31 million people passed, overnight, to being considered hypertensive, largely increasing the contingent of individuals eligible for chronic anti-hypertensive prescription. A study published in the *Journal of the American Medical Association* details how this decision drastically expanded medication consumption without necessarily offering clinical benefit proportional to the new contingent.

This type of diagnostic expansion, often justified as "prevention," carries a dangerous distortion: by treating as pathology what was previously a functional or adaptive variation of the organism, or even failing to focus on sustainable long-term actions, medicine creates entire markets for interventions that, in another context, would be considered unnecessary, while not decreasing pathology incidence in the population. It is an exercise in futility. The desire to place the body within an ideal statistical range overrides, in diverse cases, consideration of the impact of this choice on the patient's life.

Male sexual dysfunction is an interesting case of this logic. Previously understood as a multifactorial and relational phenomenon, with emotional and social roots, it was transformed into a clearly delimited clinical entity, treatable with standardized medications. The popularization of sildenafil (better known by the trade name Viagra) reconfigurated the definition of the dysfunction itself. The medicine created the diagnosis, not the other way around. Sexuality, instead of a field of experience, became a performance protocol. The global market for erectile dysfunction drugs is predicted to pass US$ 3 billion in 2025 to approximately US$ 6.74 billion by 2034.

Ivan Illich had already anticipated this movement in *Medical Nemesis* (1975), when he coined the concept of "cultural iatrogenesis": the tendency of medical institutions to redefine daily life in clinical terms, creating dependence on offered solutions (without, ironically, generating more health). According to him, the greatest risk was the medicalization of existence. Disease became not only treatable but mandatory, because it was the passport of access to the legitimacy of suffering—and to its profitability.

The exponential growth in the number of psychiatric diagnoses in recent decades—driven by successive editions of the *Diagnostic and Statistical Manual of Mental Disorders* (DSM)—does not necessarily correspond to an increase in disorder prevalence, but to the expansion of their categories and criteria. Between DSM-IV and DSM-5, there was a quantitative and qualitative leap in classifications, which came to include increasingly tenuous, heterogeneous, and socially modulated conditions. Disorders like ADHD, generalized anxiety disorder, and mild depression began to be diagnosed en masse, often based on isolated reports, standardized in rapid questionnaires, and treated immediately with recurrent high-cost medications.

Now, look how intriguing: a study published in 2012 in *PLOS Medicine* revealed that 69% of the panel members responsible for drafting DSM-5 maintained financial ties with the pharmaceutical industry. This data compromises the scientific independence of the world's most influential manual in mental health, and also raises an uncomfortable question: how many of the diagnoses justifying continuous pharmacological treatments today were defined under direct influence of economic interests and without broader treatment? Psychiatry, which should be a space of listening, context, and integral care, has become, in many cases, a field of automatic prescription and industrialized labeling.

Meanwhile, the structure of reimbursements and health systems reinforces this cycle. In countries with public systems, like Brazil, the logic is adapted in the form of forced productivity: doctors pressured to see dozens of patients per shift, with 10 or 15-minute windows for each consultation. Listening, in this model, is simply unfeasible. When plans remunerate by volume and complexity, but not by clinical result or well-being, perverse incentives are created that feed the institutionalization of disease, and even countless frauds, which end up being a major problem for insurers paying for unnecessary and often unexecuted procedures.

Recent reports from the National Supplemental Health Agency (ANS) show an expressive increase in complaints related to procedures charged but not performed, or excessive prescriptions aimed at profit and not clinical necessity. Health procedure fraud alone causes a multi-billion deficit for the entire ecosystem. Value-based remuneration models have been proposed as an alternative, but their implementation still runs up against deeply ingrained regulatory and cultural structures.

This distortion is aggravated by loopholes in the regulatory structure itself. Agencies like ANS (in Brazil) and CMS (in the US) establish coverage packages based on diagnostic categories but do not penalize the absence of outcome or the repetition of ineffective interventions. A hospital can perform dozens of exams on a patient with chronic pain without ever investigating their life history, and still be fully remunerated for each of these acts. The system thus rewards the persistence of the symptom, not its understanding. And this reward, dear reader, does indeed configure a conflict of interest.

We are talking about a historically constituted, economically sustained, and culturally naturalized phenomenon. Facing it requires more than denouncing—it demands unveiling, with clarity and depth, the gears maintaining a model that transforms failure in the mission of promoting health into a business. Denouncing this is rescuing what it should be: an instrument of care, of potency restitution, of life amplification. The critique of disease institutionalization does not deny the importance of technique, pharmacology, or technology. But it demands that all of them subordinate themselves to the question: does this favor life? And this subordination, my dears, should be non-negotiable.

THE PROFITABLE CYCLE OF DEPENDENCE

The healthcare system sustains itself financially with sick people. Not those who die, but those who remain sufficiently sick to return. This logic, although rarely stated explicitly, permeates decisions, remuneration models, research investments, and institutional design. Recurrent disease has become, for many market players, more profitable than the cure.

This distortion begins in the financial heart of the system we already cited: the fee-for-service model. A *Health Affairs* study revealed that US hospitals obtain, on average, 86% more revenue from patients who return within 30 days after discharge than from those who recover permanently. In other words, relapse is more profitable than resolution. This logic, handed over to business people, is a feast for actions of dubious ethics.

In Brazil, the logic reproduces similarly in large health plans, especially those operating under accreditation regimes. The provider is incentivized to see as many as possible in less time and prioritize quantity over quality. In 2022, ANS recorded that 71% of complaints against plans involved difficulties in accessing continued treatments or coverage denial, a clue that the focus is more on cost containment than care transformation.

The patient, then, neither heals nor cares for themselves; they return. Not because the doctor consciously desires this, but because the entire ecosystem drives them in this direction. Anti-hypertensives are ingested daily by millions of people for decades. The same goes for metformin, statins, bronchodilators, and serotonin reuptake inhibitors. The relief is immediate. The dependence, too.

And here is a neuralgic point: many of these drugs were tested and approved for prolonged use, but without the industry proportionally investing in research for regeneration, remission, or reversal of conditions. The cycle feeds itself. In 2019, the *Journal of the American Medical Association* published an analysis showing that 72% of investments by major pharmaceutical companies were directed at chronic control therapies and not disease eradication. The strategic focus? Conditions of high recurrence, low mortality, and long therapeutic permanence.

This logic reinforces itself in the field of psychiatry, where the medicalization of complex emotional states has become the rule and long-term psychotherapy the exception. It is estimated that more than 50 million people worldwide have been on continuous antidepressant use for over five years—without a clear discontinuation plan, without a reintegration strategy. The industry, by offering rapid relief, transformed feelings into syndromes whose solution are pills and recommendations without commitment.

Studies from the Cochrane Collaboration (the world's largest organization dedicated to preparing and maintaining systematic reviews of the effects of health interventions, itself already involved in corruption and conflict of interest allegations) indicate that guidelines with indirect sponsorship are 4 times more likely to recommend continuous and pharmacological treatments than those with an independent base. 4 times. 400% more likely. Wait, do we have a problem here?

Despite exponential advancement in biotechnology, genomics, and personalized medicine, large-scale initiatives aimed at regenerative interventions, evidence-based integrative practices, or metabolic re-education are rare. This is not so easy to monetize. In contrast, there are hundreds of studies to develop new analogues of already profitable drugs, a kind of "incremental innovation" that, fundamentally, renews patents and prolongs revenue chains.

An emblematic case was the opioid scandal in the United States. Purdue Pharma, maker of OxyContin, hid data indicating the drug's dependence potential for years. By promoting it as safe for chronic pain, it created an entire generation of dependent patients, and a multi-billion dollar prescription market. The episode revealed how continuous profit can also be leveraged by side effects of the solution itself. This same pattern, on a different scale, can be identified in areas like dermatology, endocrinology, gastroenterology, and so on.

It is even more serious when this logic disguises itself as prevention. The marketing of palliative preventions (exams generating more exams, supplements promising what they don't deliver, or corporate health programs producing an infinity of exams and monitoring without intervening) creates an illusion of self-care, which, in practice, expands control (and revenue) without transforming the outcome.

At the other end, the SUS (Brazil's Unified Health System) suffers from unresolved chronicity. Data from DATASUS show that 78% of ambulatory visits in primary care are related to conditions like hypertension, diabetes, and musculoskeletal pain. A good part of these cases could be prevented or reversed with regenerative care models, but scarce funding, team fragmentation, and absence of transversal care lines prevent this. The disease remains, and the queue grows. Faced with this, it is impossible not to raise a fundamental ethical question: what if the current system is functioning exactly as designed? What if the problem is not its dysfunction, but its perverse efficiency?

Behind the scenes of this cycle operate financial plans frequently led by those very close to who approves or rejects investments, and very far from who needs maximum efficacy in care, with a focus on "predictable return." In many cases, the success of a clinic or network is measured not by the quantity of discharges with resolution, but by the quantity of appointments and follow-ups.

There is even a geopolitical component amid this dynamic. The pharmaceutical industry represents a relevant slice of GDP in countries like Switzerland, Germany, and the United States, creating a structural economic incentive for maintaining chronicity on a global scale. Drugs like insulin, statins, antidepressants, and anti-hypertensives move billions of dollars every year. Even with the advance of biotechnology and artificial intelligence, the predominant logic of clinical research still favors continuous symptomatic treatment.

Curiously, the idea that "continuous treatment is better than cure" has naturalized to the point of becoming consensus. Many professionals do not even realize they are operating within this logic. After all, everything seems to work: patients return, exams follow one another, symptoms are controlled. Disease becomes manageable, but a triad of profound side effects exists: the first is the corrosion of hope of no longer having the disease. When the system only offers control, the patient begins to resign themselves. The idea of reversal, regeneration, or cure starts to sound utopian, esoteric, or "alternative." Health care as structured today, by limiting itself to control, ceases to be imagined as a path to freedom, when science shows that, often, it is possible.

The second is the atrophy of clinical creativity. When all protocols point to the same cycle—diagnosis, prescription, return—the space for listening, personalization, and therapeutic boldness narrows. And the third, perhaps the gravest, is the economic and social crisis. A system depending on disease to finance itself will inevitably become unsustainable. And the numbers already clearly show this. The explosion of chronic diseases, population aging, and pressure from judicialization are making the current model economically unviable. A McKinsey study projects that, if nothing is done, costs with chronic diseases worldwide will exceed 47 trillion dollars by 2030. No tax, health plan, or incremental innovation can sustain this curve.

For all this, it is urgent to recognize: the current health system is in crisis because it functions exactly as designed. And this design, founded on disease recurrence, needs to be reviewed. By naming the cycle of dependence, we can begin to break it. And for this, more than our good intentions is needed: incentives must be redesigned, regenerative practices financed, education for reversal established. Profit can then come from this new dynamic, from value generation aimed at more quality of life and regeneration. It's a lot, right? But all this is already happening, popping up around the world more and more—and artificial intelligence is exponentially accelerating this curve. Much of what we see today will be unthinkable in a few years, just as the scope of the health professional and physician will transform along with it.

THEMATIC FOCUS: WHY THE SYSTEM PREFERS PATIENTS WHO ALWAYS RETURN, BUT NEVER GET TOO BETTER

✦ Pharmaceutical Industry

- How it profits from continuous illness: Revenue from chronic and recurrent medication use, especially for symptom or partial biochemical control.
- Evidence: Pfizer and Novartis profit far more from chronic diseases (e.g., hypertension, diabetes) than from spot cures. (IQVIA, 2023)

✦ Health Plans

- How it profits from continuous illness: Charge premiums based on projected risk, but operate under a logic of controlled loss ratio—not health promotion.
- Evidence: McKinsey study (2021) shows plans invest less than 5% of revenue in primary prevention.

✦ Hospital Systems

- How it profits from continuous illness: Paid per procedure and admission. The more recurrence and chronicity, the higher the occupancy and billing.
- Evidence: Fee-for-service models still predominate in most countries, including US, Brazil, and much of Europe.

✦ Standardized Clinical Protocols

- How it profits from continuous illness: Prioritize reimbursable, replicable, and rapid conduct, even if poorly personalized.

- Evidence: Guideline-based care is easier to audit, but not necessarily more effective for complex diseases. (BMJ, 2019)

✦ Labs and Exams

- How it profits from continuous illness: Bill from frequent screenings, standardized panels, and routine check-ups, even without symptom or clear benefit.
- Evidence: Mass check-ups move more than US$ 50 billion per year globally. (Global Wellness Institute, 2022)

✦ Healthtech Startups Focused on Monitoring

- How it profits from continuous illness: Many monetize data without robust interpretations, and constantly monitored biomarkers for control, creating behavioral dependence in anxious users.
- Evidence: Wearable companies profit more from users who monitor obsessively than from those reaching balance or better habits.

✦ Regulatory Agencies

- How it profits from continuous illness: Often captured by corporate interests, approve therapies based on surrogate metrics (e.g., biomarker reduction, not functional improvement).
- Evidence: Peter Gøtzsche denounces the phenomenon of regulatory capture in various books and papers. (BMJ, 2014)

✦ Traditional Medical Education

- How it profits from continuous illness: Trains professionals focused on disease control.

- Evidence: 85% of medical schools have no structured curriculum in preventive medicine. (Lancet Commission, 2020)

WHILE CURING IS A SPOT ACTION, CHEAPER AND RESOLUTIVE, KEEPING THE PATIENT UNDER CHRONIC MANAGEMENT GUARANTEES CONTINUOUS AND PREDICTABLE REVENUE, WHICH IS THE STRATEGIC OASIS OF ANY COMPANY PARTNER, WHERE ONE BILLS ON RECURRENCE. THE ENTIRE STRUCTURE—FROM CONSULTATION TO HOSPITAL—WAS DESIGNED TO OPERATE UNDER A FLOW OF CONTROLLED SYMPTOMS (VERY DIFFERENT FROM "HAVING MORE HEALTH") FAVORING THE PROFITABILITY OF MOST HEALTHCARE COMPANIES TODAY. MEDICINE CENTERED ON ILLNESS IS PROFITABLE, AND WE CANNOT FAIL TO CRITICALLY LOOK AT THIS DYNAMIC, NOR NEGLECT ITS EFFECTS ON THE ENTIRE HEALTHCARE MARKET. HEALTH, SO FAR, HAS NO BUSINESS MODEL.

A HEALTHCARE SYSTEM NOT DESIGNED TO CURE

Information relevant to patient safety remains invisible to those needing it at the most decisive hours, and little evolution can truly be built with technology and Artificial Intelligence without first integrating the data representing different snapshots of the patient's situation. Algorithm learning, to truly produce intelligent and precise answers, uses large volumes of data as input. The more incomplete the learning database, the worse the AI answers will be and the more limited its performance. True intelligence is not built, much less on a complex subject like health, full of vectors influencing it.

In many institutions, reducing the average time per consultation is considered an efficiency gain. This conflict between decisions benefiting the short versus long term is a complex dichotomy affecting any company, and here it is no different. Partners, investors, managers pressing for defensible efficiency in financial planning and management. And on this seesaw, when there is no clarity on the advantage of being more strategic in the long term, or a leader who is a guardian of quality and the broader vision of impacts and consequences of offered care, the "financism" wanting to "maximize revenue" without a strategy behind it usually wins the battle—even when this means invisible financial loss over time (invisible, mind you, because no one managed to measure it, or because these impacts do not present themselves immediately).

The most alarming part is that this entire operational and institutional arrangement is frequently presented as neutral or technically inevitable. Rare are the managers who recognize they are facing a political and economic engineering of care, where every indicator, every service flow, and every timing decision embeds moral and strategic choices. And these choices, historically, were made not to favor cure or regeneration, but to manage disease, contain legal risks, and guarantee financial predictability—fundamentals of any business, yes, but here applying to a market whose object is not just any product, but human life.

Some institutions are, in fact, redesigning their systems based on principles of integrality, continuity, and bond. Value-based healthcare models have demonstrated it is possible to organize services remunerating the patient's sustainable improvement. Clinics like Iora Health and HealthPartners in the United States, and national experiences like that of Hospital Israelita Albert Einstein, have tested approaches where listening time is protected, teams are multidisciplinary, and the patient journey is treated as a continuous process.

These initiatives remind us that design matters. The way a health service is structured—from office configuration to remuneration logic —defines not only the patient experience but also clinical efficacy and the dignity of professionals' work.

What often goes unnoticed is that the system design itself shapes clinical reasoning: patients with complex complaints are pushed into 15-minute slots in scheduling and digital triage systems; electronic medical records prevent narrative entries. In the current logic, it is easier to schedule an MRI than to get a consultation with time for expanded listening. The imbalance between diagnostic technology and relational technology is a hallmark of the disease-oriented model.

Even when the professional wants to escape this logic, the system makes it difficult. Clinicians dedicating themselves to listening and careful construction of explanations are often warned, pressured, or penalized for "not meeting expected productivity." Listening becomes a risk. Deep care is perceived as inefficiency, and the result is a silent and generalized burnout among the best professionals, who watch the erosion of their vocation under a flood of questionable goals that, sooner or later, culminate in burnout.

"Clinical journey design," a concept molded from design thinking applied to health, shows that every patient experience is shaped by invisible micro-decisions: how reception is done, how much time before interruption, who speaks first, what language is used, whether there is legitimate space for doubt or not. Today, these decisions are almost always determined by productivity, not relational clinical effectiveness.

Some innovative experiences in integrative medicine, in the US and Germany, have been testing co-consultation models, where the patient is listened to by more than one professional simultaneously. This allows summing visions, building more complete narratives, and synchronized interventions exiting the common fragmented relay. Reports show increased diagnostic precision, greater patient involvement, and clearer, shared clinical decisions.

In Brazil, Hospital Israelita Albert Einstein and Hospital das Clínicas of University of São Paulo (USP) Medical School have multidisciplinary teams collaborating in co-consultations to integrate different specialties coordinately. In China, Beijing Traditional Chinese Medicine Hospital and Guangzhou Integrated Medicine Hospital exemplify the combination of traditional practices and modern Western medicine, with a holistic approach to patient care.

It is worth emphasizing: this is not about individual bad faith (in most cases). Most professionals, managers, and entrepreneurs sincerely believe they are offering the best possible. The problem is systemic, structural, and cultural. And, therefore, so difficult to transform: because it is naturalized. Because it seems logical. Because it is efficient at what it proposed to do—even if that is not curing.

Finally, it is necessary to recognize that technology, although having more transformative potential than ever, has been used to consolidate this model. Electronic medical record systems, risk prediction algorithms, and telemedicine platforms, when designed without systemic vision, only accelerate the logic of maintained disease. Digital transformation, without ethical transformation and transversal vision "from the factory" or by design, loses much of what it could be and stops saving lives.

PATIENT, PROFIT, AND THE CROSSROADS OF THE NEXT DECADE

Clinical practice is at a historic inflection point: on one side, it carries the weight of a system designed to orbit disease—with its logic of recurrence, fragmentation, and continuous monetization of illness. On the other, it faces a technological revolution that, if well designed, can unbalance this mechanism and inaugurate a new paradigm of care centered on health regeneration, integrated data intelligence, and the potency of the subject who knows they need more. But this transition requires conscious choices, political decision, deep redesign of incentives, and a new clinical imaginary about what caring for health means.

For decades, technological advancement served, mostly, to intensify the pillars of this model: greater diagnostic precision, more control over symptoms. Wearable technologies made tracking biological parameters (heartbeat, glucose, sleep, steps) a daily affair. But, isolated, this data says little—they are metrics without semantics. Numbers, not narratives. Instead of a leap in meaning, what was seen was the digitization of the same logic that sickens: the hypertrophy of monitoring dissociated from context.

The question, then, is not whether we will have more data, but which data—and for what. Technology can favor autonomy, prevention, physiological regeneration, and reconnection with the diverse factors influencing our health, but it won't do so if those developing it lack this focus. A platform today automating prescriptions can, with another design, facilitate active listening, personalized triage, and clinical reasoning oriented to human complexity. What matters and needs to be questioned and widely validated is the intention embedded in the tool's architecture.

Models like Virta Health in the United States have been demonstrating it is possible to promote type 2 diabetes remission with structured nutritional education programs, continuous remote support, digital guidance, and individualized adjustments, using technology as a transformation catalyst. Instead of prescribing insulin indefinitely, the model bets on dynamic monitoring and behavioral change. Data is integrated and read together with life context. The result: patients ceasing to be perpetual customers to become protagonists of their regeneration.

Integrative medicine clinics have used generative AI as an extension of clinical listening. Natural language interfaces are trained to also harvest emotional states, habits, family bonds, and biographical trajectories. Technology organizes this information into intelligent reports amplifying consultation quality and preparing the ground for the bond.

This type of approach is being called *Context-Aware Clinical Conversational AI*. The term is still recent, but already appears in publications and startup prototypes combining natural language, semantic processing, and integration with biomedical knowledge bases; the differentiator lies in its capacity to incorporate subjectivity, ambiguity, and biographical context as part of clinical reasoning for expanded listening and professional resolution power.

Studies like *A Systematic Review of Context-Aware Digital Behavior Change Interventions to Improve Health*, published in *Translational Behavioral Medicine* (Oxford Academic), reinforce this model's efficacy. Context-sensitive digital interventions produce greater adherence, more consistent clinical results, and sustained emotional engagement. Diverse other studies continue expanding this field, exploring how personalization based on contextual data can potentiate patient involvement and clinical decision precision.

Simultaneously, platforms emerge betting on remuneration models for sustained health, not isolated medical acts. An example is the Cityblock Health system, aimed at vulnerable populations in the US, combining home visits, mobile technology, longitudinal medical records, and multidisciplinary teams with integral health goals. Professionals are paid to keep the patient out of the hospital, not to fill them with exams. The logic reverses. Profit comes from health—not disease.

The health system implemented in Singapore with the HealthHub platform also moves in this direction. It focuses on a financing model based on sustainable health outcomes, integrates patient health data into an electronic medical record accessible to both professionals and users, and promotes self-care and prevention. The system incentivizes robust primary care practices and proactive chronic disease management, and health professionals are evaluated and remunerated based on population health goals, such as reducing avoidable hospitalizations and effective control of chronic conditions.

In Brazil, initiatives betting on integrated regenerative protocols begin to stand out. Examples include Hospital Israelita Albert Einstein, developing preventive health programs based on integrated laboratory data and continuous monitoring. What these experiences reveal is that the future will not be decided by technical innovation alone, but by the purposeful design of systems. And this is the key point we want to bring here: either we place the patient as the center of potency, or we continue aggravating the crises of healthcare ecosystems.

Technology carries the intentions and priorities of who designs it. What does it mean, then, to "care" when having access to real-time data, predictive algorithms, and integrative models? It means deepening the capacity to see the patient before they fall ill, respecting the body as a complex ecosystem and not a simple machine, making the consultation a meeting of shared intelligence, not a repetition of prescriptions.

But, let us not be naive, this transformation is not smooth. Major players still operate under the dependency paradigm. Startups are pressured by investors to show growth based on recurrence and not resolutive impact. Professionals fear appearing "alternative" or "idealistic" when proposing regenerative practices. And patients themselves, often, have been so conditioned to the control model that they mistrust the idea they can heal and even directly ask the doctor for the medicine prescription.

In this new scenario, artificial intelligence has a central role, not as a substitute for clinical reasoning, but as its profound ally. An AI understanding nuances, structuring listening, orchestrating data with meaning. Trained with life stories, not just laboratory exams. Validated by integral health outcomes, auditable, sensitive to each patient's social, emotional, and environmental context. In sum, an ethical, integrated, and regenerative AI by design.

In the next chapters, we explore in more depth how this regenerative logic can be implemented in protocols, systems, platforms, public policies, and clinical flows. But, for now, what matters to make clear is that the fork in the road is already happening in front of us. Technology can continue promoting disease as a business model or can inaugurate a new model combining science, care, and regeneration.

And this choice is not technical.

THEMATIC FOCUS: WHAT IF PROFITING FROM HEALTH WERE THE MODEL?

✦ Definite Clinical Discharge

✘ How it profits from continuous illness: Revenue loss from procedures and returns.

✓ In a pro-health system: Shared savings model: the institution is benefited with part of the savings generated by not re-admitting the patient in 12–24 months (e.g., ACOs in the US).

✦ Chronic Disease Control with Habit Change

✘ How it profits from continuous illness: Reduction in medication consumption, consultations, and monitoring.

✓ In a pro-health system: Clinics or health teams receive bonuses for "sustained functional outcomes" (e.g., glycated hemoglobin controlled for 12 months with non-pharmacological intervention).

✦ Reduction of Unnecessary Exams

✘ How it profits from continuous illness: Drop in lab revenue and mass billing.

✓ In a pro-health system: Bonus for "efficient diagnostic precision": fewer exams with greater clinical accuracy, traceable via outcome auditing (e.g., value-based medicine).

✦ Hospital Discharge Without Readmission

✘ How it profits from continuous illness: No systemic stimulus to guarantee stability after exit.

✓ In a pro-health system: Financial reward linked to zero readmission targets at 30, 90, and 180 days (like the bundled payment model of Medicare/Medicaid in the US).

✦ Prevention of Avoidable Diseases

✘ How it profits from continuous illness: No direct remuneration; effort is seen as "cost" to the provider.

✓ In a pro-health system: Public or private financing linked to population results (e.g., drop in childhood obesity, smoking cessation, health programs in neighborhoods, schools, universities, and institutions).

✦ Effective Dehospitalization of Complex Cases

✘ How it profits from continuous illness: Reduction in hospital stay length generates less billing.

✓ In a pro-health system: Bonus based on "days of life at home without adverse event"—model proposed in various primary care innovation centers.

✦ Doctor Integrating Knowledge and Coordinating Care with Systemic Vision

✘ How it profits from continuous illness: Underpaid and considered less technical.

✓ In a pro-health system: "Health manager physician" model with bonus for "360" performance (e.g., composite indicators: adherence, bond, well-being index, key biomarkers) and competitive remuneration.

✦ Patient Who Does Not Return Because They Are Stable and Functional

✘ How it profits from continuous illness: Drops off the system radar; does not generate recurring revenue.

✓ In a pro-health system: Enters as a "traceable success case," generating performance scores in value payment platforms (e.g., QALY - Quality-Adjusted Life Year-Based incentives. QALY is a standard for measuring how treatments improve patients' lives and is used in cost-effectiveness analyses).

✦ Non-Pharmacological Interventions (Mindfulness, Nutrition)

✘ How it profits from continuous illness: Rarely reimbursed, even if they work.

✓ In a pro-health system: Integrated into multiprofessional care bundles with cross-financing (e.g., "Health Homes" and integrated initiatives in Scandinavia).

A health system that thrives on true health demands more than good intentions. It demands new remuneration models, long-term indicators, valorization of the clinical bond, and institutional courage to reward those who resolve, not those who merely administer the disease. What seems utopian is, in fact, a matter of architecture and political will. But what many have not yet understood is that when disruption establishes itself with viability and generates value for the consumer market, the entire market transforms—the old tends to be extinguished or shrunk, while the new appear and gain hegemony all over the world as the "new possible".

CHAPTER 6
CHECKUP: THE PLACEBO OF SELF-CARE

THE IMAGINARY OF THE CHECK-UP AS SELF-CARE

The check-up today occupies a place of symbolic prestige in medicine. It is, without a doubt, a valuable technical achievement: a structured protocol of exams and evaluations that, when well indicated, allows for the identification of silent alterations and generates objective data for clinical follow-up. For at-risk populations, with relevant family history, established comorbidities, or occupational exposure, the check-up can be decisive. And, in contexts marked by care negligence or low health literacy, it represents an entry point for screening subclinical diseases. It is a potent instrument. And it is precisely because of its potency that it becomes so urgent to examine it with critical attention: what was meant to be a clinical screening tool has transformed, culturally, into an artifact of control and an illusion of self-care.

In its modern origin, the concept of the check-up as a "care package offer" emerged in the United States in the 1920s, as an attempt to reduce work absences and disease costs among employees of large corporations. Over time, driven by health plans, private hospitals, and the technological evolution of diagnostic medicine itself, the check-up gained an aura of obligation. It went from an occupational health screening protocol to a kind of personal responsibility rite: those who "take care of themselves" get check-ups. Those who don't are being sloppy or irresponsible. This silent moralization of bodily surveillance changed society's relationship with care. What should be a technical instrument, situated within a larger clinical context, became an annual rite of passage—detached from the patient's history.

The multiplication of executive check-up packages, marketed as experiences of sophistication, status, and safety, shows the consolidation of a market that feeds on anxiety and the illusion of control. Large private hospitals in Brazil and the world began offering check-up services with gourmet coffee, executive transport, personalized welcome kits, private rooms, home collection, and reports bound with institutional visual identity, as if the aesthetic experience could compensate for the preventive superficiality of these exams. It is the luxury of diagnosis as a ritual of belonging to an elite that can anticipate illness, even if, often, it does not prevent it.

The growth of this sector is expressive. According to a survey by Grand View Research, the global market for personalized check-ups exceeded 48 billion dollars in 2022 and is expected to grow at a rate of 8.5% per year until 2030. In Brazil, the largest private hospitals in São Paulo, Rio de Janeiro, and Brasília already offer packages exceeding R$ 15,000, with variations ranging from genetic assessments to sophisticated cardiometabolic mappings, even for young and asymptomatic people. The offer is based on the ability to pay for more exams, more screens, more images—in a logic of diagnostic accumulation that, in practice, transforms health outcomes very little.

The critique here is not against the check-up as a resource. It is against its transformation into a substitute for prevention. Doing routine exams is very useful in various situations. But this does not equate, under any hypothesis, to an effective preventive process. Prevention acts before the risk takes shape, alters habits, acts on lifestyle, questions contexts. The check-up acts after deregulation has already begun, and is, therefore, a form of early screening, not structural prevention. The confusion between these two layers—screening and prevention—is one of the central distortions of today's medical-social imaginary.

This distortion is fed by a culture that sees isolated numbers more than complex reasoning. It is the stamp of approval that the body is "in order." Private hospitals sell exam packages not as clinical investigation, but as a wellness product. What is sold is peace of mind, and the check-up thus becomes a high-prestige emotional placebo.

Instead of paying attention to their sleep, their diet, their stress, their bonds, or their internal signals, the person learns to look at the paper that determines if "everything is right." When the numbers fit into the infamous reference ranges, even in the face of fatigue, anxiety, or imbalances, the person feels cleared to continue at the same pace, as if the body hadn't said anything. The check-up is absolution. It is the return to the comfort of statistical normality, even when the body cries out for change.

Studies have already documented this limitation. A publication in *BMJ Quality & Safety* (2014) concluded that routine check-ups in asymptomatic adults are not consistently associated with a reduction in overall mortality. In 2021, an analysis by the *New England Journal of Medicine* reinforced this: exams can detect diseases in early stages, but the impact on life expectancy is limited. Furthermore: the psychological and physical harms of false positives and unnecessary procedures can be significant. The phenomenon of overdiagnosis is today one of the great dilemmas of mass screening.

In Brazil, the check-up market has grown in recent years also as a product of social differentiation. Executive packages, which include everything from a private driver to gourmet meals and individual suites, are sold by large hospitals as exclusive experiences. And, in this scenario, the subject is led to believe that, by performing this annual ritual, they are anticipating disease when, in practice, they are only monitoring if it has already begun to set in. True prevention—which would require rethinking routines, habits, bonds, environments—remains out of the equation (or in timid and unstructured recommendations that serve almost as a protocolary ✓). The patient begins to trust the result more than their own bodily perception. Health becomes a PDF file looking like an evaluation: "Very good, you passed! All levels within normal limits!"

Health professionals also suffer the effects of this logic. Many find themselves pressured by patients to request exams even without clear clinical indication. And, faced with punitive judicial systems and a culture of professional defense, they end up giving in. The check-up becomes a poorly grounded defensive practice. And, in this cycle, the medical consultation is emptied: instead of investigating the patient's trajectory, listening to their story, exploring habits and social determinants, the doctor becomes a dispatcher of off-the-shelf exams.

This may be useful in some situations, but it is tragic as a dominant model, because it downgrades the patient's singularity, ignores contexts, and functions as a containment frame. And that is why it is urgent to reclaim the value of the check-up within a broader vision of care. It can indeed be an entry point, an attention trigger, a powerful tool, but never a substitute for the process of clinical listening, bond building, understanding habits, and supporting life change. It cannot continue to be sold as prevention, when in practice it is, in most cases, a limited corrective screening.

SCREENING CONFUSED WITH PREVENTION

First of all, it is important to remember the differences between levels of health attention and assistance in Brazil. Primary care aims to prevent the appearance of diseases, promote health through vaccination, healthy habits, and control of risk factors. Secondary screening focuses on the early detection of conditions before they become more serious, using screening exams and check-ups to identify diseases in early stages. Finally, tertiary screening reduces the impact of an already established disease, seeking to minimize its complications and improve the patient's quality of life with treatments and rehabilitation.

The check-up is not a primary prevention strategy. At most, it acts as secondary screening. But the way it has been promoted by companies, health systems, private plans, and even campaigns masks this essential distinction. The subject is led to believe that, by doing an annual blood collection, a routine CT scan, or an electrocardiogram, they are "taking care of their health" and preventing diseases. They are not.

The problem with this confusion is that it shifts the population's behavior to a comfort zone based on the illusion of anticipation. Instead of the focus being on transforming habits, eating better, sleeping with quality, taking care of mental health, and maintaining an active physical routine—all proven to be related to the prevention of chronic diseases—the system invites the patient to "track their numbers." Preventive medicine ceases to be the construction of potency and becomes a search for potential failures.

And this deviation is well documented. In 2019, the U.S. Preventive Services Task Force revised its recommendations on routine exams and highlighted that the "annual check-up" for asymptomatic adults, without risk factors, has marginal benefit and can even generate adverse effects such as overdiagnosis, unnecessary anxiety, and low-value procedures. A study conducted in Japan in 2021, published in the *Journal of General Internal Medicine*, analyzed data from more than 50,000 individuals subjected to regular check-ups, and concluded that standardized routine exams in healthy adults resulted in a 15% increase in unnecessary medical interventions, including biopsies and treatments for conditions that would not evolve into significant health problems.

In Brazil, a survey by the Ministry of Health, released in the report "Guidelines for Prevention of Chronic Diseases" of 2020, highlighted the importance of prevention strategies based on individual assessment and contextual factors. The study revealed that programs focused on behavior change, such as the promotion of physical activity and healthy eating, had a more significant impact on the reduction of chronic diseases compared to mass routine exams. The recommendation was clear: prevention is done with an individualized approach, behavior change, health promotion, and intervention on social determinants. But, instead of pushing for structural public policies (such as healthy eating, active urban spaces, reduction of ultra-processed foods and pesticides, and health education), it suffices to "keep exams up to date."

Large hospitals and operators have assembled veritable catalogs of exams segmented by age, gender, socioeconomic profile. Many of these packages include high-cost exams with low clinical indication, such as MRIs without justification, complete genetic panels, tumor markers that serve no purpose for general population screening, and laboratory analyses disconnected from the patient's history. 34% of exams done in routine check-ups lacked clear clinical justification nor impacted therapeutic changes in a relevant published study.

Entire health systems are burdened by this inefficient model that waits for the body to have an alteration before acting. Data from the Institute for Clinical and Economic Review show that, in the US, up to

27% of total costs with laboratory exams stem from screenings with no clear clinical value.

In Brazil, while the SUS struggles to offer resolutive primary care and regular consultations, large private networks sell check-up packages as a strategy for loyalty and market differentiation. The patient is induced into a consumerist behavior: they do not seek a life change, but an annual validation of their normality (recurrence once again present here without clear value delivery). And when something appears in the exams, there is no structured longitudinal network to welcome the finding in an integrated way.

Evidence that this model is ineffective accumulates. The review published in the *Cochrane Database of Systematic Reviews* (2019) concluded that annual "health checks" do not reduce mortality from cardiovascular causes or cancer in asymptomatic adults, and even increase the number of unnecessary diagnoses and treatments. A study conducted in South Africa, published in the *South African Medical Journal* (2020), demonstrated similar results that annual check-up programs in urban populations had no significant impact on reducing overall mortality, but increased the detection of clinical conditions of little relevance to patient prognosis.

Research conducted in China and released in the *Chinese Journal of Preventive Medicine* (2021) pointed out that annual check-ups in asymptomatic adults resulted in a considerable increase in excessive diagnoses, without clear benefits in reducing chronic diseases over time. Prevention, according to the authors, depends on health education, balanced diet, smoking cessation support, regular physical activity, restorative sleep, and bonding with multiprofessional teams—actions we all know are definitive for someone's health, but which are rarely stimulated or monitored by conventional check-up packages.

The challenge, therefore, is to resignify it. Stop selling it as a substitute for prevention and reposition it as part of a broader care process. This implies reviewing policies, remuneration models, and also educating the population to recognize that the absence of alterations in the exam does not mean the presence of health. And that true prevention begins in daily life. And those who propose to care for people's health need to seek means, tools, technology, and methods to influence the patient in these vectors. It is not easy—if it were, we would not have the global health crisis we have—but the intention and coordinated work to build these solutions to foster effective forms of prevention is already happening.

RESCUING PREVENTION AS A PRIORITY

The idea of prevention needs to be rescued from the semantic hijacking it has suffered. For decades, it was transformed into a euphemism for "early detection." In practice, what is called prevention, especially in commercial models, is nothing more than an anticipation of diagnosis. This is valid in some contexts, but cannot be confused with true preventive work: that which acts before the problem exists, modifying the factors that make it probable. And it is precisely this conceptual confusion that sustains the modern check-up industry.

The problem is treating the exam as an emotional shield, while maintaining habits that lead, silently, to the path of chronic disease. The body continues accumulating inflammation, stress, sleep deprivation, social disconnection, and excessive glycemic load, but "laboratory normality" produces a false sense of immunity that inhibits prevention.

Breaking this cycle requires resignifying what we call preventive care. This starts by understanding that prevention is behavior, bond, environment, and context. It is not enough to identify the problem early; one must transform the terrain where it is born—and health professionals need to enter this circuit (we know, it's not easy). And this involves literacy in risk factors, motivation for change, longitudinal support, access to health-promoting environments, and clinical presence capable of activating the desire for transformation. All of this is systematically absent in the current check-up model. That is why, despite all diagnostic advances, chronic diseases do not stop growing. This equation is not that complex; it is just deeply rooted, which causes, in many of us, a feeling that this is what is possible.

Integrative clinics have been abandoning fixed exam packages and adopting solutions based on real risk profiles, combining spot exams with deep clinical interviews, emotional analysis, lifestyle data, and artificial intelligence. Instead of delivering a static report, these initiatives offer care proposals in continuous construction.

Some healthtechs are proposing even more disruptive formats.

There are already platforms using artificial intelligence to calculate dynamic risk of illness, based on environmental data, reported habits, and emotional markers captured in real time. The focus shifts to identifying deviations from the functional health axis and intervening before the body breaks. The exam ceases to be a starting and finishing point. It becomes a tool, among several, in a longitudinal care journey.

The Chinese company Ping An Good Doctor integrates AI into its platform to assess health risks dynamically and combines user behavior data with environmental and public health information. In the United States, the startup Ginger uses AI to monitor emotional markers and offer mental health support in real time. In Brazil, the healthtech Laura developed an AI system that early identifies clinical deteriorations in hospitalized patients to reduce risks and be more proactive in patient health management.

To offer a synthesis of these contrasting layers, we present below a comparison with three existing check-up models. This comparison does not intend to hierarchize rigidly, but to illustrate the different prevention paradigms coexisting in today's scenario:

THEMATIC FOCUS: 3 CHECK-UP MODELS AND THEIR CARE LOGICS

Target Audience

- **Mass Check-up (Classic):** General population.
- **Premium Check-up (Executive):** Top executives and urban elites.
- **Emerging Integrative Models:** Elites and niches.

Selection Criteria

- **Mass Check-up:** Age + institutional routine.
- **Premium Check-up:** Ability to pay.
- **Emerging Integrative Models:** Risk profile + lifestyle.

Exam Type

- **Mass Check-up:** Standardized fixed packages.
- **Premium Check-up:** Sophisticated and detailed exams.
- **Emerging Integrative Models:** Personalized exams with clinical basis.

Consultation Approach

- **Mass Check-up:** Rapid, technical, and superficial.
- **Premium Check-up:** Cordial, but focused on exams.
- **Emerging Integrative Models:** Expanded clinical interview + active listening.

Context Analysis

- **Mass Check-up:** Rarely included.
- **Premium Check-up:** Spot and technical.
- **Emerging Integrative Models:** Central to the care model.

Technology Use

- **Mass Check-up:** Traditional laboratories.
- **Premium Check-up:** State-of-the-art equipment.
- **Emerging Integrative Models:** Dynamic algorithms + data integration.

Temporal Focus

- **Mass Check-up:** Spot and static evaluation.
- **Premium Check-up:** Diagnostic predictability.
- **Emerging Integrative Models:** Adaptive longitudinal monitoring.

Effect on Health

- **Mass Check-up:** Almost null in the long term.
- **Premium Check-up:** High chance of overdiagnosis.
- **Emerging Integrative Models:** Behavioral and environmental intervention.

Main Risk

- **Mass Check-up:** False positives and omissions.
- **Premium Check-up:** Diagnostic iatrogenesis and anxiety.
- **Emerging Integrative Models:** Low adherence due to required initial effort.

Most chronic illnesses are silent, multifactorial, progressive, and no spot exam is sufficient to intercept this trajectory without a longitudinal listening of the body, mind, and context. True prevention demands more, even if the tools and methods to exercise it at the potential it brings today are still scarce, technocratic, or poorly grounded.

Finally, it is necessary to return to prevention its meaning: *pre-venire*, "to come before." And coming before, here, is detecting before, understanding before, caring before, listening before. It is creating systems, practices, and relationships capable of acting in the field of the possible before the inevitable happens. Prevention, in this sense, is first and foremost a way of being with the patient, not a package of exams.

THEMATIC FOCUS: INTEGRATIVE AND PERSONALIZED CHECK-UPS AROUND THE WORLD

Paracelsus Klinik Lustmühle (Switzerland)

- **What they do differently:** Complete evaluation based on biological and functional medicine. Includes cellular toxicology, microbiome, environmental screening, and bioresonance.
- **Adopted model:** Integrative medicine with focus on deep causes and mitochondrial detoxification.

The Center for Innovative Medicine (USA)

- **What they do differently:** Focus on prediction and prevention through genetic, metabolic, epigenetic, and environmental analyses.
- **Adopted model:** Personalized medicine, epigenetics, and dynamic prediction.

Next Health (USA)

- **What they do differently:** Offers genetic panels, complete hormonal screenings, biological aging (age testing), and lifestyle analysis, with individual plan.
- **Adopted model:** "Bio-optimization" and personalized longevity, with AI.

Klinik St. Georg (Germany)

- **What they do differently:** Combines clinical exams with integrative oncology, deep immunological evaluation, heavy metal and parasite analysis.

- **Adopted model:** Environmental medicine and integrative oncology.

Biosalud Day Hospital (Spain)

- **What they do differently:** Integrates regenerative, autoimmune, and functional medicine in check-up programs for reversal of metabolic dysfunctions.
- **Adopted model:** Biological medicine and advanced detox.

Clinique La Prairie (Switzerland)

- **What they do differently:** Longevity and rejuvenation program: includes molecular profile, genetic sequencing, microbiome, and cellular medicine.
- **Adopted model:** Luxury preventive medicine based on translational science.

These centers approach listening, science, and systemic interpretation with integrated data, multiple layers of analysis, and personalized clinical design. They are examples of practical rupture with the fragmented model of the traditional check-up, and still largely inaccessible.

CHAPTER 7
THE BUREAUCRACY THAT SICKENS THE CAREGIVER

THE BUREAUCRATIZATION OF CARE IN THE AGE OF ELECTRONIC HEALTH RECORDS

The healthcare system also sickens its professionals by replacing care time with documentation, workflow, and reporting time. Administrative overload dehumanizes clinical practice, hollows out the vocation, and generates severe illness among an entire army of frontline professionals.

For centuries, care was grounded in listening, direct observation, and the relationship of trust between the one suffering and the one caring. Bureaucracy, when it existed, was minimal: brief notes made as memory aids, not legal requirements. The physician's legitimacy came from experience and problem-solving, not procedural codes. With the advancing institutionalization of medicine, especially from the 20th century onward, this scenario was reversed. The doctor-patient relationship began to be mediated by administrative structures, procedure tables, clinical guidelines, health insurance plans, and, more recently, digital platforms. The consultation, once guided by narrative, became anchored in forms and systems. Medical practice was gradually reconfigured as a cog within a regulatory, financial, and legal apparatus that demands ever more records, protocols, and proof, even if it comes at the cost of presence and listening.

The reality for thousands of professionals is marked by an overload that has little to do with *health* or *care*. According to a 2022 survey published in the *Journal of General Internal Medicine*, primary care physicians in the US spend two-thirds of their time on bureaucratic tasks: filling out charts, responding to messages, requesting authorizations. In Brazil, the situation is similar, especially within private health plans, where the multiplicity of operators and rigid rules impose a routine of obstacles and rework.

This loss of focus compromises the quality of care. Exhausted professionals, pressured by productivity targets and drowning in inefficient systems, have less mental and emotional space for what really matters: listening, thinking, caring. And this pressure reaches far beyond doctors. Nurses, psychologists, physical therapists, and other frontline professionals report high levels of burnout related to excessive documentation. In nursing, the time spent on records in many Brazilian hospitals occupies up to 40% of the workday. And often, these are redundant records aimed at institutional protection or legal compliance.

The mantra fueling this model is well known: "If it isn't documented, it didn't happen." While relevant in safety contexts, this principle has transformed into a dogma that imprisons the clinical act. Everything must be recorded, but not to build a complete reading of the patient. The professional transforms into an occurrence typist, not a therapeutic agent.

Digitization has not solved—and in many cases, has aggravated—the problem. A Harvard Medical School study showed that the average time to fill out an electronic health record (EHR) can consume more than 16 minutes per patient, even when the consultation lasts only 20. Instead of freeing up time for care, technology has hijacked it. And the most alarming and ironic part is that many of these systems were designed to meet the requirements of insurers and hospital accounting. The doctor fills in mandatory fields, codes symptoms, and awaits authorizations. The digitized system has become a production line with the aesthetic of innovation.

The judicialization of medicine has intensified this movement. The fear of lawsuits leads many professionals to practice so-called "defensive charting": long, standardized notes written for protection. What should be evidence of a clinical bond becomes defense documentation. And the patient notices. Patient experience surveys show that the sensation of inattention weighs heavier than a difficult diagnosis.

Another limiting effect of this model is the standardization of the clinical narrative. Many electronic health records reduce the possibility of free or broad descriptions of symptoms and contexts, prioritizing drop-down lists (with pre-defined categories), closed menus, and structured fields. Clinical practice, which has always been an art of interpretation and listening, is reduced to a basic database.

The emotional impact is profound. Many professionals report losing the pleasure of attending to patients. They feel more like data entry clerks than caregivers. And this daily frustration, repeated in silence, sickens just as much as any grueling shift. This is what is known today as *moral injury*.

This scenario repeats itself worldwide. In various countries, medical associations have mobilized to denounce excessive bureaucracy in the practice of medicine. In the United States, the American Medical Association launched the "Fighting Physician Burnout" campaign, pointing to digital bureaucracy as a leading driver of exhaustion. In the United Kingdom, the Royal College of General Practitioners has pushed for reforms that return consultation time and clinical autonomy to family and community doctors. In South Africa, the South African Medical Association has highlighted the impact of bureaucracy on the quality of care, especially in rural areas where a lack of resources is compounded by complex administrative processes. In India, the Indian Medical Association has raised concerns about the increased administrative workload compromising time dedicated to direct patient care. In Germany, the Marburger Bund, the hospital doctors' union, has campaigned to reduce excessive paperwork and increase the efficiency of hospital systems.

The challenge of bureaucracy in medicine is a global issue requiring solutions adapted to different contexts and realities. By taking center stage, bureaucracy undermines care, the professional, and patient health, and indirectly but forcibly drives up costs for the entire ecosystem by rendering it consistently less effective.

It is also worth emphasizing: this type of effect (where bureaucracy and administrative objectives are inflamed within operations) is extremely complex to perceive, measure, admit, and tackle by companies in any sector. The entire institutional apparatus (including guidelines, leadership and partner decisions, regulations, and business models) puts down such deep roots in the *modus operandi* that it *becomes* the operation itself. Dismantling it to reassemble it (even for the better) is perceived as a "painful" change with high costs, prioritized only when there is an urgent or force majeure situation that almost induces mobilization. Anyone who has lived through a "simple" replacement of an ERP, CRM, or back-office system understands this point well. And here, we are talking about something more complex than systems. You know the story of the frog that boils if placed in a pot of cold water that is heated slowly? We are in that pot, burning ourselves without realizing it.

However, there are reaction movements. "Slow medicine" proposes a more deliberate clinical practice centered on connection and listening. Clinics like Iora Health (USA), now part of One Medical/Amazon, or Kry (Sweden) have restructured workflows to reduce bureaucratic burdens and put technology back at the service of the relationship. But for this, one must have the courage to ask the right questions: Why do we record so much? Who does this record serve? What intelligence is produced with it? Recording is necessary—but only if the documentation serves the care, not the other way around.

That is exactly why this chapter exists: before we talk about everything we can create with what technology allows us today, we need to place a magnifying glass on where we are chronically dysfunctional, with institutionalized deviations of purpose that brake or even prevent health-focused innovations. We need to redesign care so that the healthcare professional can be an agent of transformation. This requires time, structure, training, and culture. But above all, it requires the courage to recognize that a system that sickens those who care compromises everyone's health and is condemned to fail.

If medicine wants to rediscover its regenerative power, it will need to free itself from the bureaucratic labyrinth that currently imprisons it. This means placing records or protocols at the service of life—and not the machine.

THEMATIC FOCUS: ANATOMY OF BUREAUCRATIC EXHAUSTION

How the system designed the caregiver's fatigue

Remuneration by volume and procedure (fee-for-service)

⛓ ***How it manifests:*** Pressure to increase the number of appointments per hour.
⚠ ***Consequence for the caregiver:*** Loss of bond with the patient, superficial service, burnout from "production."
✱ ***What should occupy this space:*** Remuneration models based on outcome, connection, and resolution (value-based care).

Digital systems built without clinical listening (complex EHRs)

⛓ ***How it manifests:*** 70% of consultation time spent filling out mandatory fields.
⚠ ***Consequence for the caregiver:*** Reduced listening time, feeling like a "healthcare clerk."
✱ ***What should occupy this space:*** Clinical interfaces that support reasoning and liberate care.

Insurance and payer audits with a purely financial focus

⛓ ***How it manifests:*** Denials of procedures, rigid protocols, interference in conduct.
⚠ ***Consequence for the caregiver:*** Ethical frustration, therapeutic impotence, loss of medical autonomy.
✱ ***What should occupy this space:*** Clinical evaluation based on context and professional technical judgment.

Judicialization and the culture of punishment

⛓ ***How it manifests:*** Defensive conduct, excessive testing out of fear of error.
⚠ ***Consequence for the caregiver:*** Illness from institutional paranoia, constant fear of being punished.
✱ ***What should occupy this space:*** Culture of mutual trust, integrated legal training, and collective review of errors.

Non-human productivity indicators (time, number, "efficiency")

⛓ ***How it manifests:*** Metrics like "average consultation time" or "fill rate."
⚠ ***Consequence for the caregiver:*** Blaming those who try to listen, rewarding those who fragment.
✱ ***What should occupy this space:*** Indicators centered on patient well-being and integral outcomes.

Fragmentation among professionals and lack of dialogue between teams

⛓ ***How it manifests:*** Task redundancy, rework, low continuity of care.
⚠ ***Consequence for the caregiver:*** Fatigue from lack of coordination, demotivation with the structure.
✱ ***What should occupy this space:*** Integrated teams, protected time for case discussion, and horizontal listening.

Excessive forms, checklists, and low-utility protocols

⛓ ***How it manifests:*** Professionals forced to follow steps with no clinical value.

⚠ ***Consequence for the caregiver:*** Disconnection from purpose, sensation of sterile automatism.
✱ ***What should occupy this space:*** Living, adaptable protocols that respect clinical singularities.

Bureaucracy in health is an active vector of illness—designed to protect structures, not people. What started as quality control and fraud mitigation became a system of surveillance, productivity (complete with financial bonuses to health plan employees for denying procedures—often in life-or-death cases), and standardization that transforms caregivers into administrative operators.

FROM MEDICINE TO DATA ENTRY: THE COLLAPSE OF CLINICAL PRACTICE

The bureaucratic burden falling on healthcare professionals is an old phenomenon, but its current intensity directly compromises the original meaning of clinical practice. Every year, the volume of documents, authorizations, reports, and administrative tasks that doctors and care teams must fill out, review, or justify increases due to regulatory, contractual, or institutional demands that have little dialogue with patient well-being. This reality, frequently erased from official discourses on care quality, is today one of the central axes of caregiver illness.

This accumulation of tasks was potentiated by the digitization of health systems. The electronic health record, which promised integration and time savings, ended up, in many institutions, becoming a labyrinth of mandatory fields, redundant alerts, and rigid workflows that capture the professional's attention and distance them from the patient.

In Brazil, data from the Federal Council of Medicine and the São Paulo Medical Association indicate that doctors, especially in the SUS (Unified Health System), deal daily with fragmented systems, unintuitive interfaces, and multiple layers of simultaneous demands. In many Basic Health Units, the same encounter must be entered into two or three distinct systems: one for the municipality, another for the Ministry of Health, and another for internal control. Doctors seeing over 20 patients a shift, needing to record every detail in different platforms and still justify procedures to operators and auditors, have no mental space to sustain an attentive, reflective, and compassionate clinical practice.

All this bureaucracy interferes directly with professional autonomy. Many protocols impose mandatory sequences that stifle clinical judgment. Medicine approaches the assembly line, and care becomes a technical script that allows no deviation. This phenomenon has a special impact on primary care, where listening and bonding are the pillars of resolution. When a family doctor's schedule anticipates 10 appointments in four hours, with requirements for complete chart filling, updating preventive programs, electronic prescribing, and generating statistical reports, the space to think *about* and *with* the patient disappears. Care becomes a task, and the task becomes exhaustion.

It is a sum of invisible tasks: multiple logins, guide authorizations, duplicate entries, document tracking—which, together, consume hours of the workday without any direct contribution to care. A 2023 Medscape survey pointed out that American doctors spend, on average, 15.5 hours per week on non-clinical activities.

In Brazil, the effects of this machinery are aggravated by technological precariousness and team overload. In many contexts, especially in the SUS, systems still require manual entry or face frequent instability. There are basic health units where the internet signal is intermittent, forcing professionals to record data on paper to digitize later—rework that further reduces the time available to care. Bureaucracy adds to precariousness, and precariousness becomes part of bureaucracy.

Nurses, psychologists, nutritionists, physical therapists, and community health agents are also dragged down by documentary requirements, quantitative goals, and operational workflows centered on management. What should be a multidisciplinary team acting in an integrated manner often communicates via spreadsheets. Multidisciplinarity becomes managerial theater. The consequence is an organizational culture that values those who "hit the target." More thorough professionals, who avoid unnecessary medicalization or dedicate more time to the patient, are penalized with overloaded schedules, productivity demands, and veiled criticism for "straying from the standard." Greater effectiveness, my dear reader, is penalized, and this is extremely grave.

This inversion of value generation is the fruit of a logic that contradicts its main objective. The desire to organize, monitor, and standardize the system transformed into a tangle of requirements that swallows care time and drains professional energy. The more one seeks to control the system at any cost and without the intention of seeing the patient's journey and outcome, the less space remains to care for people.

THE BROKEN PROMISE OF DIGITIZATION: WHEN TECHNOLOGY GETS IN THE WAY

Digitization in health emerged as a promise of relief: to reduce the weight of bureaucracy, expand access to clinical data, facilitate communication between professionals, and, above all, return time to care. But the reality in a good part of healthcare systems is different. The introduction of digital technologies, especially electronic health records, failed to deliver these benefits and, in many contexts, worsened overload, increased the distance between doctor and patient, and distorted the logic of care. Instead of bringing closer, the screen began to mediate and, in many cases, to impede.

The electronic health record is an emblematic case of this unfulfilled promise. Created, in theory, to organize clinical information and reduce redundancies, it became, in practice, a recording system aimed at billing. Mandatory fields are designed to ensure reimbursement and satisfy audits, and the healthcare professional finds themselves forced to navigate through dozens of tabs, menus, and checkboxes in an unproductive choreography that often steals time from looking, listening, and being present.

Beyond the excessive time consumed, there is the problem of cognitive fragmentation. Many EHR systems force the professional to enter information out of the logical sequence of a consultation. Symptoms go in one tab, history in another, physical exam in a third, conduct in a fourth, prescription in an integrated external system (when integration exists). This fragmentation interferes directly with clinical reasoning. As Donald Schön, philosopher and MIT professor of urban planning, warned, professional thinking is deeply influenced by how we record and organize information.

Interoperability, another great argument for digitization and indeed a fundamental condition for evolving the vision of everything that affects health, also remains far short of what was promised. Most hospital systems and clinics still operate with proprietary software that does not communicate with one another. The result is a patchwork of digital scraps where patient history gets lost. The doctor at one hospital cannot access exams done at another. The emergency room does not see the clinician's notes. In 2017, a Joint Commission study in the United States revealed that lack of access to complete information was a contributing factor in 80% of serious adverse events analyzed. The information exists—but it is in another system. Once again, the number is worrying.

The issue lies in the design, incentives, and objectives that guided the construction of these systems. As Professor Atul Gawande warned in his article "Why Doctors Hate Their Computers," published in *The New Yorker*, health systems adopted technologies designed for administrative control. In interviews conducted in the UK and published by the *British Medical Journal*, doctors reported that they began avoiding eye contact with patients for fear of delaying typing into the system. Some even develop tendonitis from excessive mouse and keyboard use. Others report that, at the end of a shift, they must spend hours "closing cases" (not with the patient, but with the system).

A Canadian Medical Association report showed that 63% of professionals interviewed consider electronic health record systems a factor in increased stress, and 47% said it negatively impacts their relationship with patients. Why, in a sector as sensitive as health, were digital systems built with so little empathy for the user? Part of the answer lies in the structure of the health technology market itself. Many systems were designed by companies focused on administrative demands. The logic of compliance overrode the logic of care.

Another relevant factor is the absence of co-design with frontline professionals. Instead of involving health professionals and patients in system creation, many solutions were imposed from the 'top down,' in purchasing processes led by financial managers, legal teams, and purchasing committees that usually evaluate the non-financial impacts of a choice superficially. Technology was treated as a commodity. And the result was predictable: systems designed without attention to usability, with artificial workflows and languages that do not dialogue with clinical practice.

In many countries, health digitization was promoted as a panacea—a universal solution for all the sector's ills. Public policies invested billions in computerization, often without adequately preparing professionals or evaluating the impact on care. Digitization became a buzzword and a goal in itself.

In 2015, the NHS (UK health system) launched the "Paperless 2020" program, promising to eliminate paper in public hospitals. The project was widely criticized for prioritizing administrative goals without resolving integration, usability, or data overload problems. In 2018, the project was reformulated, with less focus on digitizing for the sake of digitizing, and more attention to the professional experience. In Brazil, *Conecte SUS* was announced as the integrating platform for all citizen clinical data. The idea was ambitious and quite interesting: to unify histories, reports, vaccines, and prescriptions. But implementation hit infrastructure problems, lack of a single standard between systems, and low adherence by municipalities. In practice, a good portion of professionals still depends on manual notes or disconnected local records.

Experiences demonstrate that, when well-designed, technology can expand care. AI pre-triage tools have saved clinical time. Speech-to-text software, transforming doctor's speech into text during consultation, already shows good results. Systems integrating clinical data with social and behavioral variables have improved chronic patient management. The problem is the adoption model.

The central question is: who is technology serving? The patient? The clinician? The manager? Or the finance department? When digital solutions are born from listening to practice, mapping functional workflows, and co-construction with users, the result is different. Technology stops being a barrier and becomes an ally. And, it must be made very clear: Finance and Purchasing teams, in a healthy corporate structure, must submit to strategic decisions that make sense for generating business value, not the other way around—precisely to avoid decisions that are seemingly financially advantageous but deteriorate what is non-negotiable in the long run and compromise an entire ecosystem (and lives, and the business itself).

To advance more quickly in this, a profound redesign of digital workflows will be necessary. Instead of requiring the professional to fill out dozens of fields, why not use AI to suggest automatic fills based on history and context? Instead of forcing navigation through rigid tabs, why not allow a narrative interface, with freedom to write, organize, and connect information logically, which intelligence will help structure? Instead of imposing identical systems for everyone, why not allow intelligent customizations by specialty, clinical profile, and context of action?

The startup Suki AI, which we have already cited, uses voice commands to allow doctors to make clinical notes while talking to the patient and has shown a significant reduction in typing time. Notable Health automates administrative tasks with AI, freeing professionals for what really matters. The Hospital das Clínicas in São Paulo, in partnership with USP, developed interoperability solutions based on FHIR (Fast Healthcare Interoperability Resources), a global standard allowing more efficient and secure data exchange between different platforms.

With the advancement of conversational AI, such as OpenAI's ChatGPT and Google's Gemini (among many others), which are increasingly being integrated into platforms and software, we can already see a trend of these tools supporting individuals in interpreting exams and diagnoses. Today, it is already possible, within the Google platform (Docs/Drive, email), upon accessing a file, to automatically access Gemini's interpretation of the document, including exam reports. The issue is leading digital back to its original role: to facilitate, to empower. Technology needs to be gentle with the professional's time, respectful of the patient's time, and an ally of clinical reasoning.

THEMATIC FOCUS: INITIATIVES THAT IMPROVED THE CLINICAL EXPERIENCE

Suki AI (USA)

Artificial intelligence platform that uses voice commands to transcribe clinical notes in real-time.

➤ *Impact on clinical practice:* Significantly reduced time spent on documentation, allowing doctors to focus more on patient care.

Meu SUS Digital (Brazil)

Evolution of public health system *Conecte SUS*, integrates patient clinical data, including medical history, exams, and vaccines, accessible by professionals and citizens.

➤ *Impact on clinical practice:* Improved continuity of care and reduced redundancies, promoting a more holistic view of the patient.

Delta Bots (Brazil)

Startup from Minas Gerais, Brazil, developing AI and automation solutions to optimize administrative and clinical processes in local health units.

➤ *Impact on clinical practice:* Increased operational efficiency and improved quality of care, especially in resource-limited communities.

Clinical Pathways (UK)

Visualization and flowchart tool aiding doctors in diagnostic evaluation for clinical decision support.

➤ *Impact on clinical practice:* Facilitated clinical data analysis, improving decision-making and efficiency in diagnosis and treatment.

LIVO (Spain)

Platform connecting hospitals to nursing professionals using AI to optimize schedules and work reconciliation.

➤ *Impact on clinical practice:* Increased professional flexibility and improved human resource allocation, reducing professional burnout.

THEMATIC FOCUS: INITIATIVES THAT AGGRAVATED CHALLENGES IN CLINICAL PRACTICE

Fragmented Electronic Health Records (global)

Non-integrated EHR systems with complex interfaces.

⚠ *Impact on clinical practice:* Increased administrative load and reduced time available for direct patient care.

Conecte SUS (initial versions) (Brazil)

National platform that faced interoperability and usability challenges in its initial versions.

⚠ *Impact on clinical practice:* Hindered efficient access to patient information, negatively impacting continuity of care.

Accelerated Digitization Programs (UK)

Initiatives like "Paperless 2020" implemented without proper co-design with health professionals.

⚠ *Impact on clinical practice:* Generated frustration among professionals due to lack of alignment with real clinical needs.

My Health Record (Australia)

National EHR system that faced public resistance and low initial adoption due to communication and privacy failures.

⚠ *Impact on clinical practice:* Many professionals reported difficulty of use and doubts regarding the reliability of inserted information.

Epic Systems (USA)

Widely adopted in American hospitals but criticized for its complex interface and steep learning curves.

⚠ *Impact on clinical practice:* Increased screen time and reduced human contact in care, contributing to clinical burnout.

Integrated Health System (Peru)

Attempt to unify public medical record systems without adequate digital infrastructure.

⚠ *Impact on clinical practice:* Resulted in instability, data loss, and clinical workflow disorganization in remote areas.

Hospitales Digitales (Chile)

Hospital digitization project with excessive focus on infrastructure but little professional training.

⚠ *Impact on clinical practice:* Created a gap between technical modernization and clinical practice, generating dependence on constant external support.

Forced adoption of unregulated healthtechs (India)

Professionals were pressured to adopt private platforms for telemedicine without standardization or training.

⚠ *Impact on clinical practice:* Generated disparities in quality of care, legal insecurity, and overload from ill-adapted systems.

THIS SELECTION SHOWS THE IMPORTANCE OF DEVELOPING AND IMPLEMENTING DIGITAL HEALTH SOLUTIONS THAT ARE USER-CENTRIC, CO-DESIGNED WITH PROFESSIONALS, AND ALIGNED WITH REAL CLINICAL NEEDS. TECHNOLOGY MUST BE AN ALLY IN CARE, NOT A BARRIER TO BE OVERCOME.

THE PAIN OF THE CAREGIVER: BURNOUT, ABANDONMENT, AND MORAL INJURY

Various frontline professionals have been facing, with increasing frequency, an exhaustion that goes beyond physical tiredness—it is an existential collapse. It is the feeling of being present but absent; of acting with technical competence but without potency; of following protocols with precision but with one's heart outside the room. This is what international authors have called *moral injury*: the pain of knowing what would be best for the patient but being unable to offer it due to constraints of time, system, structure, or budget.

A survey by the São Paulo Medical Association revealed that 57% of doctors reported emotional exhaustion, while 40% showed clear signs of professional burnout. And it is not just fatigue: many described feelings of uselessness, depersonalization, and loss of meaning in the profession. In the US, more than 63% of doctors reported symptoms of burnout after the pandemic, an alarming number that lays bare the emotional and institutional collapse of care.

This suffering is fed by a structure that demands, standardizes, clocks, and drains, without returning emotional support, protected time, or recognition. Medicine, which has always demanded intense personal dedication, began to demand superhuman performance from professionals in exhausting shifts, with multiple simultaneous demands, impersonal goals, and growing bureaucracy. The result is the flattening of the clinical professional into an administrative avatar, an executor of conduct, with no time or space to metabolize the impact of their decisions.

Burnout, here, is only the visible symptom of a profound misalignment: the detachment between the ideal of care and the reality of practice. Professionals who entered medicine to welcome and transform lives find themselves filling out forms, dealing with institutional demands, and putting out logistical fires. They feel alone, even in large teams. They feel powerless, even when technically well-prepared. They feel guilty, even when they did the best they could. And perhaps most devastating: they feel that, little by little, they are ceasing to feel. Because feeling too much in an insensitive system can be unbearable.

This tiredness strikes at identity: doctors report no longer recognizing themselves in the choices they make. Nurses, historically close to direct care, express frustration at having become operators of automated tasks, far from the listening that inspired them. Psychologists try to sustain the mental health of others while their own crumbles. The youngest, recent graduates, are faced with a reality brutally distant from the ideal that moved them: often marked by exploitation, legal insecurity, and total absence of mentorship.

And, of course, this also affects the patient. Several studies have already shown that professionals in burnout make more errors, listen less, and establish more fragile bonds. A study published in 2019 in *BMJ Quality & Safety* showed that doctors with high levels of exhaustion presented a 45% greater risk of committing significant clinical errors. The suffering of the caregiver becomes a systemic risk. The professional's pain reverberates in the quality of care and closes a cruel cycle: failure generates guilt, which feeds back into suffering, which undermines clinical potency.

This critical scenario is also expressed in the rising suicide rates among doctors. International estimates indicate that doctors have a risk between 1.4 and 2.3 times higher of suicide than the general population, especially among anesthesiologists, psychiatrists, and clinicians. In Brazil, although underreported, cases accumulate in silence. And the most tragic part is that these suicides are often not interpreted as symptoms of a sickening system, but as individual issues, personal pathologies disconnected from the structures that generated them. Pain, once again, is privatized.

But the pain of the caregiver is also multiple. There are those who suffer quietly, those who ask for leave, those who get sick in silence, and also those who resist, who denounce, who invent new practices—often against the grain. Peer listening movements, emotional decompression programs on shifts, support groups among residents, and self-managed clinics are emerging. These are genuine attempts to rescue the humanity of the practice.

What is revealed is that burnout is not just a reaction to overwork. It is a consequence of the dissociation between what the professional knows care should be and what the system allows them to do. This chasm between knowing and power, between intention and action, is perhaps the most painful place for those who chose a profession oriented toward the other. It is not the volume of hours that kills. It is the hollowing out of meaning. It is the repetition of actions that do not transform.

And this is not solved with motivational talks or mental health lectures, fruit in the break room, or slogans about "resilience." Moral exhaustion demands a moral response—collective, institutional, political, and ethical. The system needs to stop asking professionals to be heroes. And start ensuring they can be human. With time to listen, space to reflect, autonomy to decide, protection to err. And with real support networks to sustain their own health. Because there is no true care where the caregiver has collapsed. And there is no sustainable health in an ecosystem where those who care are forced to numb their emotions to survive.

THEMATIC FOCUS: DATA ON SUFFERING AMONG HEALTH PROFESSIONALS

Prevalence of burnout among Brazilian workers

30% of workers suffer from burnout syndrome, placing Brazil as the country with the second most cases in the world.

Source: National Association of Occupational Medicine (ANMT)

Burnout in medical residents in Brazil

78.4% of medical residents present symptoms of burnout.

Source: Article by Fabichak, Silva-Junior, and Morrone

Moral injury among health professionals during the pandemic

Study with 31,849 professionals in 13 countries found a moderate association between moral injury and symptoms of post-traumatic stress disorder, anxiety, depression, burnout, and suicidal ideation.

Source: Meta-analysis published in PubMed

Compassion fatigue in health professionals

Studies indicate that compassion fatigue negatively impacts caregiver health, associated with anxiety, depression, sleep disorders, and burnout.

Source: Integrative review published in Psicodebate

Burnout and moral injury in doctors

Research with doctors revealed a prevalence of 62% moderate depression, 45% moderate anxiety, 45–80% burnout, and 88% moral injury.

Source: Study published in Annals of Family Medicine

THESE DATA SHOW THAT PSYCHOLOGICAL SUFFERING AMONG HEALTH PROFESSIONALS IS A SYSTEMIC CRISIS DEMANDING STRUCTURAL RESPONSES. IT IS IMPERATIVE THAT HEALTH INSTITUTIONS, MANAGERS, AND POLICYMAKERS RECOGNIZE AND FACE THIS SITUATION AND IMPLEMENT MEASURES PROMOTING HEALTHIER WORK ENVIRONMENTS, WITH ADEQUATE EMOTIONAL SUPPORT, PROFESSIONAL APPRECIATION, AND CONDITIONS ALLOWING FOR THE PRACTICE OF TRULY HUMANIZED CARE.

THE URGENCY TO REDESIGN CARE: TECHNOLOGY AT THE SERVICE OF THE CAREGIVER

If it is true that technology contributed to overburdening and sickening those who care, it is also true that it can be redesigned as an instrument of clinical liberation. But this only happens when the logic of developing digital systems and workflows stops prioritizing billing and control, and starts recognizing time, listening, and clinical intelligence as central values of medical practice.

Experiences around the world have shown that it is possible. OpenNotes, a project created by Beth Israel Deaconess Medical Center in Boston, made the full content of clinical notes accessible to the patient. The initial goal was to strengthen transparency. But what was seen in various participating institutions was also an improvement in the quality of listening and the doctor-patient bond. Doctors began writing with more clarity, rigor, and empathy—and patients reported greater understanding, adherence, and trust.

In Brazil, the startup Phelcom developed Eyer, a portable camera with AI for automated ophthalmological screening—especially useful in remote regions. More than providing diagnoses, the system was thought out to free up specialist time, reduce repetitive tasks, and expand the resolution capacity of primary care. It is a model of technology that relieves. In Denmark, the public system implemented a unified national digital health record network, focused on interoperability. The platform connects different levels of care and allows the patient themselves to include data on their emotional state, therapeutic adherence, and lifestyle changes.

The system created by the American startup Abridge uses artificial intelligence to transcribe consultations in real-time, generate summaries in accessible language for patients, and simultaneously automatically fill in electronic health record fields. What was once an exhausting task—writing structured notes during and after the consultation—became a process mediated by technology that returns time, attention, and presence to the doctor.

Solutions aimed at the well-being of the caregiver also bring new perspectives: the *Clinician Burnout Dashboard*, created by Stanford Medicine's WELL MD Center, monitors exhaustion indicators in real-time based on system usage patterns, screen time, and self-reports of exhaustion. The logic is simple: if we monitor patients' heartbeats, glucose, and sleep, why not track the emotional vital signs of the professionals caring for them? Self-care needs to stop being an individual luxury and become institutional policy.

EmPath, a protocol applied in hospitals in the United States that reorganizes the mental health care workflow to reduce waiting times and create decompression spaces for team professionals as well, managed to significantly reduce episodes of aggression, exhaustion, and job abandonment among professionals. The most interesting part is that this redesign is more sustainable. Studies by the King's Fund, a renowned health research institution in the UK, show that initiatives reducing burnout among health professionals result in higher productivity, lower turnover, less clinical error, and higher patient adherence. Similarly, a World Health Organization (WHO) study highlights that healthy work environments reduce absenteeism by up to 25% and improve the performance of health teams.

Any technological innovation in health must be evaluated by its human impact. If a tool saves time but drains attention; if it accelerates processes but sabotages connection; if it organizes data but prevents listening—it fails and needs to go back to the drawing board. Technological success in medicine must be measured in relational health. And that includes the health of the caregiver.

This is the transition we propose: from technology as an instrument of extraction to technology as an instrument of regeneration, from the logic of blind efficiency to the logic of sensitive presence, from silent burnout to active institutional listening. And from the hollowed-out professional to the whole clinician—with time, with meaning, with health.

CHAPTER 8
THE DANGERS OF EVIDENCE WITHOUT CONTEXT

Evidence-based medicine is an undeniable technical advancement, but its decontextualized use has become a clinical limitation. Protocols and guidelines gain the status of absolute truth, while clinical reasoning, context, and deep listening are devalued. This section proposes reconstructing the relationship between evidence and patient perceptions.

EVIDENCE THAT IGNORES THE INDIVIDUAL

There is no doubt that evidence-based medicine was one of the greatest advances in clinical practice. By proposing that medical conduct be sustained by consistent data, controlled clinical trials, and systematic reviews, it created a necessary antidote against outdated empirical practices, arbitrary decisions, and dangerous intuitions. Valuing evidence brought rigor, comparability, and predictability to systems previously vulnerable to guesswork and unfounded tradition.

But it also brought a relevant side effect: the risk of blind generalization. Professionals, pressured by protocols and audits, often find themselves forced to apply guideline-based conduct even when their listening, clinical reasoning, and experience indicate that a specific patient does not fit the norm. According to research with general practitioners in the

UK, 65% report frequent conflicts between protocols and their patients' clinical uniqueness, especially in complex contexts like multiple comorbidities, psychosocial suffering, or uncategorizable symptoms. In Brazil, a study by the University of São Paulo (2022) identified that 58% of primary care physicians face the same dilemma, aggravated by structural limitations, cultural diversity, and social inequality.

The heart of the matter lies in the difference between what works "on average" and what works "in this body, at this moment, with this life history." Randomized clinical trials—the evidence ideal—are excellent for demonstrating average effects in statistically controlled groups. But their transposition to the clinic runs into an elementary datum we have already addressed: no one is an average. Each patient carries a unique metabolism, affective relationships, beliefs, traumas, routines, social vulnerabilities, and material realities that radically modulate their response to treatment. Ignoring this is blindness disguised as precision.

So-called "first-order evidence" (randomized clinical trials, meta-analyses, systematic reviews) usually disregards these complex layers. In the name of statistical controllability, those with multiple diseases, those outside the target age range, those not fully adhering to the protocol, or those presenting variations challenging sample homogeneity are excluded. The result is methodologically perfect studies, but disconnected from life. As Canadian epidemiologist John Frank stated, "evidence-based medicine is excellent for knowing what works in general, but terrible for deciding what to do with a person in front of you."

The elderly, patients with rare diseases, or people in socioeconomic vulnerability are underrepresented or completely absent from the clinical trials underpinning guidelines. A 2023 FDA (Food and Drug Administration) report indicated that while African Americans represent about 13% of the US population, they make up only 5% of clinical trial participants. In elderly people with comorbidities, exclusion is even greater. And these are, precisely, the patients who most need contextualized care.

Another critical point is evidence production itself, which exists within an ecosystem of interests, pressures, and limits rarely discussed with clarity and transparency. A Cochrane Library survey pointed out that about 75% of studies on new drugs published in the last ten years had some degree of industry funding—and that these studies were four times more likely to present favorable results for the investigated product. Information sources used by professionals to make decisions carry biases that are not clear. This demands a critical reading not always present in daily clinical practice.

There is also an important methodological issue: the obsession with objectively measurable outcomes at a shallow level. In the name of statistical robustness, most studies prioritize biological markers and hard indices like cholesterol, mortality, blood pressure, while leaving out aspects like perception of well-being, vitality, functionality, emotional adherence, meaning of life, or satisfaction with care. The patient who feels worse but improves in numbers is treated as a success case.

In countries like Brazil, where cultural, social, and biological diversity is immense, the blind application of universal guidelines can be especially damaging. A protocol built based on North American studies may not apply to indigenous populations, *quilombolas*, or patients with access difficulties, low education, or precarious nutrition. Evidence medicine, without contextual listening, can become a tool of exclusion with a technical veneer.

And it perpetuates a dangerous reductionism: that everything that matters can be measured by current tools. This quantitative illusion obscures the value of dimensions like the therapeutic bond, the illness narrative, and the patient's trajectory, which is full of uncaptured data. As Annemarie Mol showed in *The Logic of Care*, care is not organized in linear guidelines, but in affective, pragmatic, fluid networks—where technical knowledge must bend to lived life.

A significant part of the scientific community already recognizes these limitations. Movements like person-centered medicine, narrative medicine, complexity science, and personalized medicine have been seeking to recompose the equation. In Canada, Australia, and the Netherlands, national guidelines already incorporate the principle that no evidence is applicable without first being adjusted to the history, values, and situation of the one being cared for. The WHO proposes *evidence-informed* practice—where science, experience, and values coexist as inseparable parts of the clinical decision.

This perspective refines rigor. Recognizing the limits of evidence is part of its ethical and intelligent use. When a professional refuses to apply a protocol because they perceive it is inadequate for that patient, this is not rebellion. It is living clinical practice and a sign of competence.

PASTEURIZED CARE AND IGNORED EXPERIENCE

The promise of evidence-based medicine was clear and powerful: use the best available data to support clinical decisions, reduce unjustified variations in care, and improve patient outcomes. But what is seen, in every corner of Brazil, is the distortion of this promise by a rigid, decontextualized, and mechanized application of the idea of science. What was born to support clinical reasoning has converted, in many contexts, into a substitute for it, transforming the consultation into a box-checking ritual where the protocol imposes itself over listening and the guideline suffocates the singularity of the person in front.

This phenomenon, experienced by many professionals almost without realizing it, has a name: clinical checklist syndrome. A standard of care where the professional is pressured to fulfill a technical-administrative script, with little or no space to navigate the real complexities of each case. Instead of a conversation, with organic nuances and detours, a sterile sequence of predictable questions, closed answers, and automated conduct is established.

This dynamic did not fall from the sky. It is the result of a thick broth with some ingredients already mentioned, which accumulate:

1 Brutal increase in workload

2 Growing judicialization of medicine

3 Systematic pressure for productivity

4 Standardization imposed by digital systems treating care as a technical operation

5 A model remunerating by volume and punishing individuality

A patient with chronic chest pain may pass through all exams and cardiovascular risk stratification algorithms and still have their pain unexplained, or worse, labeled as "non-specific" and be referred to a psychiatrist. This disconnection between guidelines and clinical reality infiltrates from training onwards. Many students learn medicine as if it were a flowchart game. Clinical reasoning, which should be a narrative exercise of active listening and contextual synthesis, becomes a statistical scanner. And when this recent graduate falls into the real world, full of ambiguous patients, cases that don't close, bodies that don't obey, they feel unarmed, anxious, insecure.

A Stanford Medicine survey (2021) pointed out that 58% of doctors graduated less than 10 years feel their practice is increasingly distant from what they consider true care. The term most used by them? "Clinical automatism," a kind of technical torpor where the patient becomes the next number in line (you must have seen this happen a few times).

Medicine, in its essence, has always been both science and care. It demands technical knowledge, yes, but also requires presence, intuition, listening, improvisation, sensitivity. When reduced to the cold application of evidence, it loses its transforming power. And this loss has real consequences on clinical outcomes, treatment adherence, and the well-being of doctors and patients.

Judicialization also carries central weight in this collapse. Brazil, the US, and Italy are among countries where lawsuits for "not following protocol" are growing. This feeds a climate of institutional fear where care becomes defense and treatment a legal strategy. It is so-called "defensive medicine"—where more exams are ordered than reasons are heard.

This critique, once marginal, now reverberates within the community itself. Conferences, manifestos, scientific societies have been denouncing protocol hypertrophy and clinical anemia. Movements like *Realistic Medicine* (Scotland), *Choosing Wisely* (present in dozens of countries), and more humanized medical curricula seek to rescue practice as an encounter.

These movements propose a redesign of care reconciling science with sensitivity; valuing the guideline as a reference, but never a sentence; teaching the professional to read evidence as a tool; returning to the doctor the legitimacy to listen, think, intuit, and decide based on context, not just statistics or a single ineffective universal path.

WHEN CONTEXT CHANGES EVERYTHING

Consider the response to the same drug treatment among individuals of different ethnicities. Studies show that certain anti-hypertensives, such as ACE inhibitors, have reduced efficacy in black populations compared to white populations, a widely documented fact. Yet, this nuance rarely appears in rapid care protocols pointing to "the best medicine" based on statistical average, without considering ethnic, socioeconomic, or environmental variables.

The same happens with gender differences. Women often present cardiovascular symptoms considered "atypical" (like fatigue, gastric pain, or diffuse malaise) and are therefore frequently underdiagnosed in emergency care with chest complaints. The American Heart Association warned in 2022 that women are 50% more likely to receive a wrong diagnosis after a heart attack, precisely because the standard protocol was designed from studies done mostly on men.

There is also the determining role of social context in clinical effectiveness. An antidepressant with 60% efficacy in clinical trials may have a very different impact on someone living under domestic violence, food insecurity, or isolation. In these cases, the problem lies in the absence of an approach including social factors in clinical reasoning.

There are also protocols that, even if technically correct, fail ethically. A study published in the *New England Journal of Medicine* (2020) revealed that algorithms used for prioritizing patients in US health programs inadvertently favored white patients to the detriment of black patients, even when clinical indicators were similar. This is because the algorithm used past health spending as a proxy for need, without considering that black populations, due to historically limited access, spend less not because they need less, but because they are served less.

Data is generated, interpreted, and applied within systems permeated by inequalities, biases, and specific interests. And when transformed into a protocol without critical mediation, it can crystallize distortions. Statistics become, here, insufficient and unjust. The risk lies in how they are read, replicated, and applied, without listening to what escapes the numbers.

Real clinical cases help illustrate the impact of context. A patient with type 2 diabetes may have difficulty controlling her blood sugar not due to treatment disobedience, but because she lives in a "food desert," where fruits and vegetables are inaccessible. Or because she works split shifts, has three jobs, and no support network. If the protocol says "reinforce diet" or "refer to nutritionist," but context makes this unfeasible, the conduct fails even when technically correct.

An adolescent diagnosed with ADHD may actually be expressing symptoms of chronic stress, food insecurity, and domestic instability. The protocol suggests medication and psychotherapy. But if the school is oppressive, the family environment violent, and the community seized by fear, the symptom persists. Psychiatry has gradually recognized the need to include environmental, community, and historical variables in diagnostic construction.

Medical literature increasingly recognizes these limitations. Practices considered alternative seek precisely to rescue context as a legitimate part of clinical analysis. And Primary Health Care, when well-structured, has the potential to make this expanded reading, precisely because it is closer to the territory and daily life of patients.

The challenge lies in developing care models recognizing that each patient brings a body, a biography, and surroundings. That the protocol is a hypothesis, listening is a magnifying glass, and evidence without context is not science, it is reductionism.

THEMATIC FOCUS: THE 6 BLIND SPOTS OF EVIDENCE-BASED MEDICINE

What protocols ignore — and why this compromises care

Average Population as Statistical Base

- **Why it fails:** Evidence is designed based on large average samples, excluding exceptions.
- **Clinical Example:** A 42-year-old woman with autoimmune condition and intense emotional history receives standard male and ineffective conduct.
- **Plausible Alternative:** Models of stratified medicine by phenotypic and contextual profiles, not just demographic.

Rigid Exclusion Criteria in Clinical Trials

- **Why it fails:** Patients with comorbidities, psychic suffering, polypharmacy, or unstable lives are excluded from studies.

- **Clinical Example:** The evidence guiding conduct does not include patients who appear most in the SUS (Brazil's public health system).
- **Plausible Alternative:** Pragmatic studies incorporating real life variables (e.g., poverty, emotional chaos, polymorbidity).

Application of Guidelines Without Listening

- **Why it fails:** Protocols are applied like a cake recipe, without adaptation to the subject and their complexity.
- **Clinical Example:** Doctor ignores a patient's complaint because "it is not in the current guideline protocol."
- **Plausible Alternative:** Commented and adaptable guidelines with space for documented clinical judgment.

Surrogate Metrics (e.g., "reduced LDL," "improved score")

- **Why it fails:** Treating symptoms or biomarkers as ends in themselves, without looking at functional impact or well-being.
- **Clinical Example:** Patient with lower cholesterol but exhausted, depressed, and without clinical improvement.
- **Plausible Alternative:** Integrated evaluations—functional outcome, perceived vitality, restored bond.

Evidence Focused on Short Term

- **Why it fails:** Most clinical studies follow patients for weeks or a few months, not years.
- **Clinical Example:** Hormonal or antidepressant therapy seems effective in 3 months but brings complications in 2 years.

- **Plausible Alternative:** Longitudinal studies centered on sustained health, not just immediate response.

DISREGARD FOR CULTURAL AND AFFECTIVE FACTORS

- **Why it fails:** The same conduct can have completely distinct effects depending on narrative and environment.
- **Clinical Example:** Prescribing mindfulness to a woman suffering domestic violence—without listening or support—can be innocuous or cruel.
- **Plausible Alternative:** Inserting sociocultural and affective dimensions into therapeutic efficacy reading.

EVIDENCE-BASED MEDICINE WAS ONE OF MODERN SCIENCE'S GREATEST ACHIEVEMENTS. BUT THIS DOES NOT MEAN ITS METHODS SHOULD BE APPLIED WITHOUT LISTENING, WITHOUT CONTEXT, WITHOUT RELATIONAL INTELLIGENCE, AND WITHOUT KNOWLEDGE INTEGRATION ALLOWING US TO SEE THE BODY'S COMPLEXITY.

HOW TO RESCUE CLINICAL INTELLIGENCE WITHOUT ABANDONING SCIENCE

Reconciliation between science and clinical listening is already happening in diverse initiatives, practices, and research lines challenging the false dichotomy between technical rigor and human sensitivity. Medicine's own history reminds us that anamnesis, attentive listening, and careful context observation were, for centuries, doctors' main diagnostic instruments. The technological revolution brought unquestionable gains, but the error was assuming these advances should replace the clinical intelligence emerging from the patient relationship. With the AI explosion coming, this axis needs to be very well calibrated to not end up emptying the profession (protocol for protocol, AI will cost less and be more precise in many aspects, and the ecosystem will reorganize based on what is economically viable and profitable).

The person-centered medicine model proposes this reintegration and is officially adopted in countries like the UK, Canada, and Australia. Unlike the traditional biomedical model, this approach values active listening as a diagnostic tool, co-construction of the therapeutic plan, and recognition of life context as a legitimate part of clinical analysis.

Another consistent movement is narrative medicine, driven by centers like Columbia University in the US, where doctors are trained to use clinical stories as instruments of deepened listening and diagnostic elaboration. In Brazil, Primary Health Care, when practiced with quality clinical time and institutional support, shows this in practice, with evidence that municipalities with more integrated PHC teams reduced hospitalizations for conditions sensitive to primary care by up to 35%. In other words: structured listening, when applied with strategy and continuity, prevents what the protocol alone could not avoid.

This return to deepened anamnesis has also been defended by extremely relevant authors like Eric Topol, in the book *Deep Medicine*, where he proposes medicine amplified by AI but based on connection, protected time, and active listening. According to him, artificial intelligence's greatest gain will be returning to the doctor the time and attention necessary to truly listen.

In medical education, this movement also begins to appear. Harvard Medical School incorporated modules on narrative medicine, evidence-based empathy, and critical literature analysis with cultural and social lenses into its curriculum. The focus is not "humanizing" the doctor as rhetoric, but training listening as part of clinical precision. Because not every complaint fits a formal category, and many clues arise from what is not said. Because detail matters.

A NEW HEALTHCARE LITERACY: TEACHING TO INTERPRET, NOT JUST APPLY

The root of many conflicts between what science shows and clinical practice lies in how knowledge is transmitted in college corridors. Current training, even in schools of excellence, still tends to form guideline appliers rather than attentive interpreters of complexity. Scientific literacy has been reduced to a conduct booklet, and what numbers show is a generation of professionals mastering protocols but hesitating—or freezing—before what escapes the standard.

Teaching medicine, nursing, psychiatry as a translation process between evidence and each patient's individuality requires much more than good papers or updated manuals. It requires training clinicians capable of sustaining ambiguities, recognizing exceptions, asking before applying. As French epistemologist Isabelle Stengers provoked, "science that intends to impose silence on the world is not science: it is power disguised as knowledge." True clinical science asks, observes, remakes itself before what does not fit the model.

21st-century medical training urgently needs to adopt a new literacy forming critical readers of evidence. Future professionals need to be taught to detect methodological limits, sampling biases, conflicts of interest, undue generalizations. Only 37% of final-year medical students in the US knew how to correctly interpret the difference between relative risk and absolute risk in clinical trials.

Medical training, facing what AI will revolutionize in coming years, becomes less a replication technique and more a thought laboratory: a space where knowledge is interrogated, expanded, applied with criteria, and calibrated in light of patient reality, seeking data even where traditional medicine has not found it.

This new way of teaching evidence is already being rehearsed in schools adopting so-called clinical reasoning, or contextualized clinical reasoning. Students are encouraged to discuss complex cases where the guideline is confronted with patient context. The idea is not "to follow or not follow the protocol," but to understand why it may or may not make sense in that case. It is training in discernment, a skill technical medicine forgot to teach.

CHAPTER 9
THE OMISSION OF HABITS AND EMOTIONS IN CLINICAL PRACTICE

EMOTION AS A BIOCHEMICAL EVENT

Before being an abstract concept, emotion is a biochemical event. Each affective state, however subtle it may seem, triggers detectable neurochemical chains that spread throughout the organism—not only in the brain, but in peripheral tissues, organs, skin, the digestive system, the immune axis, and blood vessels, in every cell. Sadness has a rhythm, fear has a smell, anger has a temperature. Euphoria and hopelessness are equally material: both adjust receptors, alter hormonal flows, and reconfigure communication between systems such as the autonomic nervous system, the endocrine system, and the immune system. There is no "abstract" emotion. There is dopamine, serotonin, norepinephrine, acetylcholine, endorphins, pro-inflammatory cytokines, neuropeptides (and dozens of other substances whose functions are not yet fully understood), all concrete mediators of affective states that the body recognizes.

What we call "feeling" is, in fact, a complex internal signaling system. Emotions like fear or joy are embodied phenomena that mobilize specific pathways in the central and peripheral nervous systems. The limbic system, prefrontal cortex, and brainstem interact in milliseconds to interpret stimuli, issue commands, and trigger adaptive responses—

with measurable repercussions on heartbeat, digestion, immunity, and even gene expression. In parallel, peripheral tissues such as the gut, heart, and skin also participate in the reception and emission of these messages, forming a "distributed emotional system."

The literature already identifies that emotional states maintained for long periods create persistent physiological signatures capable of inducing or aggravating pathological processes. Chronic negative emotions activate the hypothalamic-pituitary-adrenal (HPA) axis and the sympathetic nervous system in a sustained manner, resulting in increased cortisol, adrenaline, and norepinephrine—stress response hormones that, in excess, alter neural plasticity, reduce heart rate variability, compromise immune function, and promote low-grade systemic inflammation.

The body interprets emotions as physiological instructions. It adjusts its functioning based on the emotional content of the experience as a central gear of its self-regulation. This chemical reading of the internal world is what makes us biologically sensitive to what we live. And it is at this point that medicine, by remaining excessively fixated on decontextualized laboratory metrics, loses an essential dimension of diagnosis and care: the meaning of what the patient lives. Without understanding this dimension, it is impossible to understand why two bodies with similar test results evolve in such different ways. The way the organism interprets, responds to, and resignifies what it feels defines the prognosis more than the exam does.

EMOTIONS THAT SICKEN OR HEAL: WHAT MEDICINE STILL HESITATES TO INCORPORATE

The idea that emotions are merely background noise, clinically irrelevant, or at best peripheral to decision-making is increasingly unsustainable. Decades of research in psychosomatics, psychoneuroimmunology, neuroendocrinology, and neuroscience have already demonstrated that specific emotional states directly modulate physiological, inflammatory, immunological, hormonal, and cardiovascular processes. Yet, what is mostly seen in healthcare continues to treat emotions as an optional add-on, to be considered if time permits. And, in practice, it almost never does.

Medicine hesitates to incorporate emotions as a clinical variable because it historically constructed itself as a field valuing objectivity. What could not be measured, classified, or isolated in a laboratory was marginalized as noise. But today, science can measure this "noise" with precision. A study from Harvard Medical School (Slavich & Irwin, 2014) shows that emotions like guilt, hostility, and fear are associated with sustained activation of the hypothalamic-pituitary-adrenal (HPA) axis, increased cortisol, and elevation of inflammatory markers like IL-6 and TNF-alpha—substances directly implicated in cardiovascular diseases, cancer, and cognitive decline.

On the other hand, emotions considered "positive," such as hope, affection, and purpose, are measurable biological modulators. The longitudinal *Nun Study*, conducted for decades in the US, analyzed a series of autobiographical letters written by nuns at the beginning of their religious lives and demonstrated that those expressing more affection and optimism lived, on average, seven years longer. A later analysis showed even lower incidence of neurodegenerative diseases, even in genetically predisposed individuals. Emotion, here, is a longevity factor.

Emotional influence on pain is also well documented. Systematic reviews published in *The Lancet Psychiatry* indicate that unresolved emotional traumas significantly increase pain perception and chronicity, especially in conditions like fibromyalgia, chronic lower back pain, and migraine. In these cases, approaches treating physical pain and emotional suffering simultaneously, such as mindfulness, cognitive-behavioral therapy, or EMDR (Eye Movement Desensitization and Reprocessing), achieve clinical outcomes superior to exclusively pharmacological treatments, but clinical protocols still ignore these interactions. Check-up forms do not ask about bonds, recent losses, psychological distress, or accumulated traumas. Cardiovascular risk spreadsheets do not include emotional variables, even when these directly affect blood pressure, heart rate, and cholesterol levels. And oncological risk scoring systems do not consider the impact of chronic stress, even though studies demonstrate its association with tumor progression.

Top hospitals worldwide are beginning to question this omission. The Dana-Farber Cancer Institute in Boston introduced a pilot protocol in 2022 for emotional assessment integrated into oncological treatment. Patients respond weekly to validated scales of mood, distress, hope, and pain, and results are interpreted alongside laboratory tests. The initiative has already demonstrated increased treatment adherence, better immune response, and lower rates of emergency hospitalizations. Kyoto University Hospital in Japan implemented an emotional care program interconnected with clinical monitoring for patients with autoimmune diseases. The protocol includes active listening practices, narrative interviews, and psychometric scales like PHQ-9 (for depression), PSS (for perceived stress), and WHO-5 (psychological well-being). The approach significantly reduced corticosteroid use and improved inflammatory indicators in patients with lupus and rheumatoid arthritis.

Resistance to including emotions as clinical data still rests on two misconceptions: first, the fear of making practice "less scientific" (revealing an outdated understanding of the subject) and, second, the supposed difficulty of operationalizing this type of data. But these obstacles today are false dilemmas. Scientific rigor already exists. And the technological tools to measure it precisely do too.

Heart rate variability (HRV) is today one of the most sensitive markers of emotional regulation and autonomic adaptability. Studies from the HeartMath Institute and universities like Stanford and McGill show that elevated HRV is associated with greater stress resilience, lower cardiovascular risk, and even better cognitive performance. Conversely, persistently low HRV correlates with chronic fatigue, burnout, and negative outcomes in various clinical conditions.

Another objective marker is salivary cortisol, whose daily curve should rise upon waking and decline throughout the day. When the HPA axis is dysregulated, this curve flattens, indicating what some researchers call "adrenal exhaustion." Correlations have already been demonstrated between this dysfunction and worse outcomes in breast cancer, treatment-resistant depression, and autoimmune diseases. Yet, this curve remains outside clinical routine.

Facial expression analysis is also consolidating as a clinical instrument. Artificial intelligence software, trained with *microexpression* databases, is already capable of identifying early signs of depression, anxiety, post-traumatic stress, and even suicidal ideation. Institutions have been developing algorithms integrating *microexpressions*, vocal intonation, and spontaneous verbal content, with accuracy superior to traditional screening.

But these technologies are still applied in a fragmented way, in pilot programs or research contexts. Institutional will to integrate them into the daily clinical system is still lacking. It is as if a barrier still separates the "emotional" from the "clinical," even with robust data demonstrating this division is artificial. And the cost of non-integration is also economic. According to the World Health Organization (2022), the impacts of chronic stress and mild mental disorders (such as subclinical anxiety and depression) generate annual losses exceeding 1 trillion dollars in productivity, absenteeism, poor therapeutic adherence, and avoidable hospitalizations.

Brazil also has initiatives pointing the way. The state government of Mato Grosso do Sul created the *Cuidar de Quem Cuida* (Caring for Those Who Care) program, focused on health professionals under emotional overload. The model includes HRV monitoring, active listening, mindfulness, and data-based psychological support. The results: lower absenteeism, greater emotional stability, and positive impacts on patient safety indicators. Another highlight is the *Hospitais Saudáveis* (Healthy Hospitals) program, coordinated by a Latin American coalition based in São Paulo, advocating for the inclusion of simple emotional markers, such as suffering scales, in chronic patient screening.

What is taking shape is a new field of action, which we could call "emotionally integrated medicine." It is not about suppressing the biomedical model, but expanding it. To include in the logic of precision not only genes and biomarkers but also emotions, bonds, and lived experience—as legitimate, traceable, and interpretable clinical data.

HABITS THAT SUSTAIN (OR SABOTAGE) CARE

Just as with emotions, the direct impact of lifestyle habits on health is widely recognized by science but rarely translates into clinical protagonism. In traditional medical practice, these variables continue to be treated as accessory elements, almost always restricted to the category of "general guidelines," given hurriedly at the end of the consultation. Instead of occupying the center of assessment, habits orbit the clinic as a prevention appendix, a "behavioral bonus" that almost never transforms into structured prescription, as if this were outside the scope. And this reinforces the paradox: what most sustains or corrodes health is present all the time but remains invisible to the dominant logic of care.

Studies from the WHO, CDC, and Harvard School of Public Health are categorical: about 80% of chronic diseases like type 2 diabetes, hypertension, obesity, dyslipidemias, and cardiovascular diseases are directly influenced by four central factors: inadequate nutrition, physical inactivity, smoking, and excessive alcohol consumption. Yet, in many clinical encounters, these factors receive less attention than a marginal variation in TSH or creatinine.

Fee-for-service remuneration models, the previously mentioned agility-based hospital flows, pharmaceutical market dynamics, and pharmacology-centered medical training contribute to habits, even if scientifically decisive, being treated as "patient behaviors" rather than measurable clinical data amenable to effective intervention.

When we analyze guidelines from respected medical associations, such as the American Heart Association, the National Institute for Health and Care Excellence, and the Brazilian Society of Cardiology, we see that guidelines explicitly mention lifestyle changes as the first line of conduct in various conditions. But in practice, clinical time rarely allows for an investigation and structured approach to these variables—much less follow-up with listening, goal negotiation, and periodic review. Patients leave with pharmacological prescriptions but without any plan to modify the daily determinants perpetuating the illness. A hypertensive patient may reduce their pressure for a few months with an antihypertensive, but if they remain sleep-deprived, under chronic stress, sedentary, and with inflammatory eating habits, the medication will temporarily mask an untreated cause.

This negligence becomes even graver in the face of evidence that well-conducted habit change can be as or more effective than medication. In 2019, the study *Lifestyle Medicine: The Evidence Behind the Six Pillars*, published in the *American Journal of Lifestyle Medicine*, demonstrated that structured approaches in nutrition, physical activity, sleep, stress management, social bonds, and rational substance use can, in various cases, reverse stable clinical conditions, such as metabolic syndrome, without the need for drugs.

Even faced with these findings, health systems have changed their infrastructures little to incorporate this type of care. One reason is the difficulty in transforming these habits into data that can be recorded, tracked, and remunerated. Research conducted by the Federal University of Rio Grande do Sul showed that general practitioners rarely note or revisit the topic of "habits" in consultations. It is as if we treated people's daily lives as irrelevant background, even knowing it is there that illness takes hold.

This erasure also explains why protocols fail so frequently in vulnerable populations, where lifestyle habits are not an individual choice but a response to the environment: food insecurity, exhausting work shifts, absence of support networks. Prescribing physical exercise without considering the individual's life logistics is repeating the blame game.

And the professional becomes uncomfortable in the terrain of behavior. Many feel unprepared or without instruments to propose lifestyle changes that sound viable, respectful, and efficient. And there is a reason for this: medical training barely contemplates aspects of behavioral change. Tools like motivational interviewing, theory of planned behavior, and health psychoeducation are still exceptions.

Therefore, international interest is gaining strength for clinical strategies transforming habits into real clinical data. Initiatives like the Mayo Clinic's Health Coach Program, the American College of Lifestyle Medicine's Lifestyle Medicine Residency Curriculum, and digital protocols applied by platforms show it is possible to prescribe, monitor, and re-evaluate habit changes with the same seriousness applied to medications.

These models utilize sensors, digital diaries, scoring systems, and automated feedback to help professionals measure progress, integrating behavioral indicators with objective biomarkers. More than "advising," these technologies structure a new type of prescription: with continuity, traceability, and measurable impact.

And when we speak of habits, we are not speaking only of conscious choices. Many behaviors are automatic responses to the environment, emotional history, family culture, and social architecture of each person's life. Thus, a realistic and clinical approach to habits needs to go beyond the discourse of "willpower" and incorporate sophisticated strategies of support, structure, reward, and daily life redesign.

There is no integral care without caring for routine, and there is no routine care without time, listening, and clinical repertoire. This demands a reinvention of various procedures, but also a mindset shift: habits are the fabric of health.

THE BIOLOGY OF AFFECTION: HOW BOND AND PURPOSE MODULATE THE BODY

Medicine is beginning, albeit timidly, to recognize what human experience has always intuited: that connection affects the body, that loneliness sickens, and that affection is a concrete physiological variable. The idea that emotions, relationships, and meaning in life modulate inflammatory, immunological, cardiovascular, and neurological processes is a consolidated field of research.

Chronic loneliness can be as harmful to health as smoking or obesity. A meta-analysis conducted by Brigham Young University, with more than 300,000 individuals, revealed that people with poor social ties have a 50% greater risk of mortality, comparable or superior to various traditional risk factors. And yet, how many times is a patient's degree of belonging explored in a common medical consultation?

A review published in *Perspectives on Psychological Science* reinforces this point: social support and emotional connection are associated with lower levels of inflammation, lower stress reactivity, and better neuroendocrine regulation, with direct impact on IL-6, TNF-alpha, CRP, and cortisol. And the study led by Steve Cole at UCLA went further: it demonstrated that loneliness alters gene expression and promotes an inflammatory pattern called CTRA (*conserved transcriptional response to adversity*). The body literally transcribes loneliness into immune activation, dropped antiviral response, and increased risk of illness.

In the opposite direction, bond and purpose increase immunoresilience. A study with seropositive patients showed that high levels of optimism and affective support were associated with lower viral load and slower disease progression. In oncology, the effect is visible: breast cancer patients with solid emotional support networks have higher treatment adherence, fewer side effects, and, in many cases, better survival—the *Social Support Intervention Trial* was a watershed in this sense. In cardiology, the data is also clear: the INTERHEART study, with more than 25,000 participants in 52 countries, identified that psychosocial factors like chronic stress and lack of support are as predictive of heart attack as dyslipidemia or hypertension.

The most intriguing part is that these effects are measurable by objective methods: functional resonance, genomic analyses, inflammatory biomarkers, and heart rate variability indices. Emotional experience can indeed be translated into objective metrics, but the health system still looks little at this. HRV has become an increasingly studied marker of integration between brain, heart, and autonomic nervous system. Low HRV, as mentioned, is associated with depression, burnout, worse post-surgical recovery, and higher mortality risk in multiple conditions —and all these states are modulated by affection and connection.

In the UK, the public health system created "social prescribing" programs where primary care physicians can prescribe activities such as listening groups, community gardening, intergenerational mentoring, and volunteering for patients with emotional suffering or chronic diseases. The goal is to strengthen real bonds as part of the treatment.

This model already shows impact on health indicators and hospital cost reduction. In Canada, the *Rx: Community* program follows a similar line, connecting patients to support networks, cultural spaces, and belonging opportunities.

In Brazil, Hospital Israelita Albert Einstein conducts studies on the impact of emotional support on critical patient recovery. In France, pilot projects have begun structuring the recording of emotional variables in clinical records, with questions about life satisfaction, family ties, sense of utility, and chronic suffering.

The impact of life purpose has also been mapped. A University of Michigan study with more than 6,000 adults revealed that having a sense of purpose reduces the risk of death in five years by 15%. In Japan, the concept of *ikigai*—the reason for living—is studied as a protective factor against neurodegenerative diseases, cardiovascular diseases, and mood disorders. The Ohsaki Cohort, with more than 43,000 participants, showed that individuals with higher *ikigai* live longer.

The challenge now is to integrate these factors into the clinic, without reducing them to motivational slogans. Today, even in advanced institutions, structured fields to record emotional aspects are still rare. At best, free notes can be made, without alerts, without analysis, without interoperability with clinical decision-making. And what is not structured is not analyzed. It gets lost in a data swamp with unstructured, untreated data unavailable for artificial intelligence. A concrete proposal would be to adopt the notion of clinical biography: an approach integrating emotional, contextual, and physiological markers. This biography would bring to light elements that exams never capture: unprocessed grief, silent guilt, chronic loneliness, feelings of uselessness —factors modulating immunity, sleep, pain, and adherence.

Psychoneuroimmunology, studying the connections between mind, brain, immune system, and endocrine system, is one of the most promising scientific bases for consolidating this vision. It studies how emotional stressors alter neurotransmitters, hormones, and cytokines (immune system messengers), with direct effects on clinical prognosis. Patients with adequate emotional support present shorter hospital stays, less analgesic use, and lower rates of post-surgical complications.

Perception of empathy in the first medical consultation is capable of reducing pain and anxiety symptoms, and improving prognosis in chronic pain cases. In mental health, this is even more evident: depressive and anxiety disorders are strongly correlated with social isolation, affective ruptures, and low perception of belonging. But even when these factors are recognized, they rarely become structured clinical data.

If a depressive condition is treated only with antidepressants, without touching the affective network sustaining or collapsing it, the risk of relapse is extremely high. Approaches like the *Circle of Security*, focused on parental bonds, or mindfulness programs, have already demonstrated impact on markers like telomeres, HRV, and interleukins (cytokines produced by leukocytes). A randomized clinical trial evaluated the use of Mindfulness-Based Cognitive Therapy (MBCT) as a complementary treatment for patients with treatment-resistant depression and showed a significantly greater reduction in depressive symptom severity and a considerably higher "response" rate compared to a control group.

TECHNOLOGIES AND LANGUAGES THAT MAKE THE INVISIBLE CLINICAL DATA

For centuries, this more subjective dimension of life was a nebulous zone of medicine—legitimate for listening, but invisible to the medical record. This scenario began to change with advances in neuroscience and digital technologies. Today, a new clinical territory emerges: the possibility of measuring the invisible. Emotional states, stress patterns, mood fluctuations, and mental variations become traceable in real time.

What previously required sophisticated laboratory tests or controlled studies can now be monitored using wearable technologies, connected sensors bringing the Internet of Things increasingly to life, voice analysis, eye tracking, and AI algorithms trained to decode affective patterns. The first leap occurred with digital biomarkers. Devices like Oura Ring and WHOOP evolved from pedometers to mobile physiological centers. They measure HRV, temperature, sleep cycles, cardiovascular load, and recovery response—all sensitive to chronic stress. Today they are used by athletes, in research on burnout, depression, anxiety, and neurovegetative disorders.

In parallel, machine learning algorithms emerged interpreting voice modulations as a mirror of emotional state. The Ellipsis Health platform analyzes 90 seconds of spontaneous speech and predicts depression and anxiety risk with over 85% accuracy, validated across diverse population profiles. Entire clinical screenings can emerge from a casual conversation.

Facial expressions also entered the radar. Combining cameras, myoelectric sensors, and artificial intelligence, companies like Affectiva and Emteq began decoding microexpressions and involuntary movements imperceptible to the human eye. Chronic pain, pediatric anxiety, suffering of sedated patients—all can now be captured as clinical data. How the gaze moves, fixes, or avoids certain visual areas can indicate specific mental states. Other discrete signals, like keystroke dynamics on mobile phones or digital navigation rhythms, are also being studied. Startup Mindstrong Health demonstrated that variations in these patterns could anticipate depressive or psychotic episodes up to two weeks in advance.

But most promising is the integrated use of these multiple sources in multimodal predictive models. Platforms like Empatica, already active in research with NASA, DARPA, MIT, and Yale, cross-reference physiological, behavioral, and contextual signals to monitor patients with epilepsy, burnout, and mood disorders in real time, with high predictive value. Beyond capturing what the patient reports, we are talking about capturing what the body reveals, even in silence. A patient with a depressive history may have their response to medication modulated by sleep indicators, HRV, and voice intonation.

The obstacle of interoperability, ubiquitous, affects here too. Most devices still operate in closed ecosystems, incompatible with public health systems or traditional medical records. Apple HealthKit, for example, which holds great potential, collects advanced emotional and physiological data but does not easily integrate with platforms like Brazil's e-SUS AB. The same occurs with Fitbit data from Google, which are not easily integrable into health management platforms and face integration barriers with systems like Epic, widely used in the US.

At the University of Toronto, the *Emotion-Aware Rounds* program trains doctors to capture non-verbal emotional signals supported by sensors and real-time feedback. The result: a 21% increase in patient satisfaction and a 12% drop in complaints about clinical communication. In Brazil, PUC-Rio studies algorithms applied to spontaneous speech in psychiatric emergencies, capable of predicting hospitalizations up to 72 hours in advance.

Most important are not the sensors, but the logic sustaining them (this is why what the reader finds here goes beyond technical didactics and functional description of initiatives and technological solutions). The human body is an affective orchestra, and illness often begins in emotional dissonances that accumulate, leaving no biochemical traces in early stages. Capturing them early is saving time, relieving suffering, avoiding costs, and unburdening the health system. And AI can be a key piece in this process to capture subtle patterns, reinforce hypotheses, and propose paths the human alone might not see. The challenge is training eyes. Forming professionals who know how to interpret emotional data with ethics, sensitivity, and clinical intelligence.

This algorithmic listening, to be effective, must be accompanied by a coherent systemic architecture. One must have the gaze that knows how to interpret this data. This is where the challenge is most complex and requires transdisciplinary practical knowledge, which is the scarcest type of scientific knowledge available. This implies reorganizing flows, training professionals, adapting medical records, and rethinking the very concept of clinical data.

Technology to measure the "invisible" already exists—what is missing is a paradigm legitimizing its use as part of clinical reasoning. And this demands a new type of professional, one understanding human complexity as an integrated system. AI can help them in this if trained beyond "micro" patterns, but in contexts, or large patterns functioning as complex neural networks suffering mutual influence. On this path, we will be closer to true health hacking, where, ideally, we can see so many factors affecting it that we can act with efficiency and anticipation never before seen in history—there will be a leap in how we treat complex conditions and chronic diseases, and this will be a great health turnaround. We will get there, but we are still far.

How the patient is received, the time given to them, the type of question, the tone of voice, body posture, are clinical devices. They modulate oxytocin release, reduce cortisol, activate trust biomarkers, and directly influence therapeutic response.

The difference between mechanical listening and emotionally intelligent listening can be the difference between capturing an early sign of dysfunction or letting it evolve until it is too late. A study conducted at Massachusetts General Hospital revealed that 60% of diagnoses of functional diseases, such as irritable bowel syndrome or chronic tension headaches, were initiated by spontaneous emotional expressions. What is called a "vague complaint" is frequently the first possible language of an ongoing systemic imbalance. Capturing it requires training and willingness to listen beyond the obvious. In Canada, the *Protected Narrative Time* pilot project experimented with a 15-minute block of free patient speech before any directed anamnesis.

Emotional language ceases to be a field of psychology or philosophy and takes its place within medicine as a science of human complexity. And emotional language is also the professional's. Professionals not trained to recognize their own emotions, not emotionally supported by their institutions, tend to replicate defensive, cold, and automated consultation models. Forming more self-aware professionals is forming more clinical doctors. Listening begins with listening to oneself, and this is neuroscience. Functional MRI studies indicate that doctors with a higher degree of emotional self-regulation activate brain regions associated with empathy and complex clinical judgment more precisely.

This finding demands a redefinition of what we understand by clinical competence. It is not enough to master pharmacology, physiology, and diagnostic logic. It is necessary to develop expanded listening, capable of reading simultaneous layers of information: symptom, affect, silence, hesitation. This listening becomes even more decisive in the most common (and most difficult) cases of contemporary clinical practice: chronic, diffuse conditions, without clear markers, but full of accumulated meaning.

THEMATIC FOCUS: TECHNOLOGIES FOR MEASURING EMOTIONS AND HABITS

Mindstrong Health

◬ **Signals captured:** Typing patterns and smartphone usage.
◍ **Physiological proxy:** Touch speed, rhythm, hesitation.
⋙ **Data interpretation:** AI models associate patterns with depression and relapse risk.
⇢ **Clinical application:** Continuous mental health monitoring.

Empatica E4

◬ **Signals captured:** Heart rate, skin conductance, temperature, movement.
◍ **Physiological proxy:** HRV, electrodermal activity (EDA), thermal changes.
⋙ **Data interpretation:** Correlation with stress, anxiety, sleep, and seizures.
⇢ **Clinical application:** Monitoring in research and clinical

applications.

WHOOP

◬ **Signals captured:** HRV, heart rate, sleep, movement.
◍ **Physiological proxy:** Heart rate as indicator of physical and emotional recovery.

» **Data interpretation:** AI models indicate physical readiness and physiological load.
⇢ **Clinical application:** Performance, stress, and recovery (including post-COVID).

Tignum

△ **Signals captured:** Adaptive questionnaires, digital behavior.
◍ **Physiological proxy:** Self-assessment crossed with cognitive performance.
» **Data interpretation:** Generation of resilience and mental energy profile.
⇢ **Clinical application:** Executive coaching and occupational health programs focused on mental agility and performance.

Biobeat

△ **Signals captured:** Vital signs via wristband (HRV, SpO2, BP, respiratory rate).
◍ **Physiological proxy:** HRV and respiratory variability as emotional and metabolic proxy.
» **Data interpretation:** Intelligent monitoring for clinical risk and stress.
⇢ **Clinical application:** Hospitals, ICU, telemedicine.

Feel Therapeutics

△ **Signals captured:** HRV, skin temperature, conductance, acceleration.
◍ **Physiological proxy:** Autonomic response to emotional events.
» **Data interpretation:** App suggests interventions based on emotional peaks.
⇢ **Clinical application:** Digital emotional therapy with wearable.

IBM Health Guardian

◬ **Signals captured:** Voice, video, text, movement signals.
◍ **Physiological proxy:** Facial expressions, speech, mobility.
» **Data interpretation:** AI microservices for depression, mobility, and cognition assessment.
⇢ **Clinical application:** Clinical research and digital biomarker development.

Welltory

◬ **Signals captured:** Physiological, behavioral, and contextual.
◍ **Physiological proxy:** Heart rate variability (HRV), heartbeats, sleep patterns, stress, and energy levels.
» **Data interpretation:** Multivariate data analysis based on HRV for stress, focus, recovery, and productivity assessment.
⇢ **Clinical application:** Non-clinical monitoring for stress management, burnout prevention, and biofeedback-based mental health support.

AutoCogniSys

◬ **Signals captured:** Daily activities, physiological signals.
◍ **Physiological proxy:** EDA, photoplethysmography (PPG), accelerometer.
» **Data interpretation:** Automated cognitive health assessment.
⇢ **Clinical application:** Cognitive health monitoring in the elderly.

Muse - Brain Activity Detection Headband

◬ **Signals captured:** Electroencephalogram (EEG), heart rate, respiration.
◍ **Physiological proxy:** Brain activity, HRV.
» **Data interpretation:** Real-time feedback for meditation and stress reduction.

⇢ **Clinical application:** Mental health and well-being.

CHAPTER 10
ENVIRONMENTS THAT SHOULD HEAL, BUT MAKE US SICK

WHAT SCIENCE ALREADY KNOWS ABOUT HEALING ENVIRONMENTS

For more than two decades, clinical studies have begun to reveal what was already obvious: the physical space where care takes place alters the patient's outcome. This finding, simple at first glance, still struggles to be recognized as legitimate clinical data. The body that bleeds or heals does not respond only to biochemical interventions, but also, and often in the most visceral way, to the noise in the hallway, the lighting of the place, the absence of windows, the metallic coldness of surfaces, the distance between the bed and the presence of someone who listens, the beeping of equipment. The environment is not background. It is an active therapeutic variable.

Evidence accumulated since the 1990s demonstrates that hospital architecture, bed design, and even the arrangement of plants in rooms significantly impact pain perception, infection rates, anxiety, and length of stay.

A study conducted by Roger Ulrich, considered a seminal landmark (*Science*, 1984), demonstrated that patients recovering from surgery who had a view of trees recovered faster and took fewer painkillers than those exposed to a brick wall. This discovery has been replicated and expanded countless times in varied contexts, but is still treated as a "cute" curiosity. Some, more skeptical, might say “great, now we need every room to have a tree in front! Very realistic!”. My most sincere answer would be: "It would be ideal - is it possible?", but it is not about that, but about understanding and putting into practice, to the extent that it can actually be done if well considered, prioritized, and with the impact well understood. And there is much more we can do besides the view with elements of nature.

The average hospital environment still seems designed to contain and monitor bodies. Even renowned institutions maintain structures that prioritize surveillance and operational efficiency above all else. The bed becomes an object of containment. Ambient sound is forgotten—or worse: neglected as inevitable noise. Lighting is standardized based on energy efficiency, often with cold spectrum lights, not on the patient's circadian rhythms. Architecture still assumes that the body is a passive object, not a sensitive entity that interacts with the surroundings.

This reductionist logic compromises the patient's experience, but above all, their healing. Scientific literature already clearly describes the relationship between environmental stress and increased inflammatory markers such as IL-6 and C-reactive protein. Natural light deprivation in long-term care environments is associated with worsening depressive conditions and greater resistance to functional recovery in the elderly. Constant noise above 60 dB—common in ICUs—is linked to sleep disorders, disorientation, increased risk of delirium, and even mortality in extreme cases.

Natural light, by itself, is a neglected medication. Chronobiology has already shown that controlled exposure to natural light during the day improves sleep quality, regulates the hypothalamic-pituitary-adrenal axis, reduces blood pressure, and even inflammatory processes. More recent studies also confirm a very strong correlation between sun exposure at sunrise and sunset and good mental health and immune system improvement. Despite this, most care environments completely ignore circadian cycle synchronization, imposing exam routines and nocturnal procedures that fragment rest and prolong illness. Studies conducted in geriatric clinics in Norway and Japan indicate that simple lighting reconfiguration, with sunset simulation, reduced nocturnal agitation episodes in patients with dementia by more than 30%. It is not little and cannot be ignored as if it were a whim.

Architecture's touch on the body is silent but decisive. Floors that reverberate noise, uncomfortable furniture, chairs that distance rather than bring closer. Space organization communicates priorities: in many offices, the computer sits between the doctor and the patient. The screen becomes the relationship mediator. The distance between patient and professional is amplified by elements that do not seem clinical but define the tone of the exchange. In pediatrics, there is evidence that the use of colors, toys, and playful settings reduces anxiety and improves treatment adherence, yet these elements are frequently treated as amenities.

Even ICUs, the epicenter of intensive care, are marked by a cruel paradox: they are high-tech, low-humanity environments, as if conciliation were impossible. Patients often remain isolated from windows, exposed to alarms and beeps that never stop, permanent strong lights, situations and possibly distressing sounds from other suffering patients in the environment, and total absence of temporal references (at most a clock hanging on the wall - which says little to the body). Research in Sweden and Canada showed that remodeling ICUs with windows, noise control, and living spaces for family members reduced length of stay by an average of 1.5 days per patient, besides significantly decreasing post-discharge delirium and anxiety.

These data should be sufficient to reconfigure architectural and clinical thinking, but awareness of this impact is quite small. When talking to health professionals about this topic, it is surprising how off the radar and agenda this is, as if it were a detail or irrelevant, which also shows, disquietingly, the level of alienation to which we are exposed. Few health systems include sensory or spatial variables in therapeutic guidelines. In contrast, so-called salutogenic architecture or salutogenic design, which proposes promoting health and well-being instead of avoiding harm (or ignoring harm caused by the space itself), is already a reality in hospitals in various parts of the world. Khoo Teck Puat Hospital in Singapore, frequently cited as one of the most advanced in the world in integrating nature, well-being, and clinical efficiency, shows it is possible to transform spaces into concrete therapeutic vectors without losing logistical performance.

More than beauty or comfort, we are talking about clinical results. A study published in 2021 in the *Journal of Hospital Administration* showed that simple interventions, such as changing colors, inserting vegetation, and reducing noise, reduced the rate of anxiolytic medication in psychiatric wards by up to 40%. Part of the resistance comes from the difficulty in measuring environmental effects, an argument echoing the same fallacy disregarding habits, bonds, and emotions in care. The subjective, here, is not the opposite of the scientific. It is what has not yet been integrated as a continuous clinical variable due to lack of technology, knowledge, or institutional decision. And this is changing. Environmental monitoring platforms in hospitals, like SoundEar (Denmark), already integrate noise levels into clinical risk dashboards. Adaptive lighting devices are already being used in Switzerland for circadian regulation. What is lacking is not technology. It is institutional will.

In many health systems, public or private, space is treated as a cost, not an outcome variable. The bed is accounted for by occupancy and average length of stay. This generates structural myopia: the cost of the blackout curtain is considered, but the cost of white light-induced insomnia is ignored. The price of a natural wood panel is calculated, but not the cost of a psychotic break in cold, reverberating psychiatric wards. Blind economy sterilizes care. The eternal dilemma between finance seeing too many costs and the need to put better elaborated and comprehensive variables into the equation repeats itself - and that is why the corporate structure, even within a clinic or hospital, needs mature leadership open to innovation, capable of expanding the care equation and inserting more complex and intelligent variables into the account. This includes the effects of readmissions, prolonged discharge times, and lower therapeutic effectiveness resulting from environmental negligence. Otherwise, my dears, the cost spreadsheet defining investments in "facilities" will accept the most convenient value for a more comfortable budget defense, and we will always be discussing what could have been and wasn't.

Even in countries with strong clinical research and innovation traditions, the physical environment is still undervalued in hospital quality indicators. Metrics like hospital infection, discharge time, reported pain, and readmission rate are rarely correlated with space configuration. This impoverishes the debate. Instead of treating the environment as care technology, it is treated as accommodation logistics, and this distinction is brutal: it defines whether the patient will be welcomed or just administered.

Curiously, sectors outside health are moving in the opposite direction. Design of corporate spaces, schools, airports, and even prisons already incorporate principles of neuroarchitecture, emotional ergonomics, and sensory regulation. Google, Apple, and Stanford University have invested for years in biophilic offices with proven impact on well-being, productivity, and burnout reduction. The same reasoning is valid—and urgent—in health.

Some reference centers are already redefining the environment as a healing agent. Maggie's Centres in the UK have cancer support centers conceived with architecture signed by names like Zaha Hadid and Norman Foster because every line, window, and texture is thought to emotionally sustain the patient during treatment. There are no corridors smelling of formaldehyde and cold lights putting anyone on alert. There are gardens, libraries, high ceilings, and silence. And clinical results appear: greater therapy adherence, lower anxiety levels, and better quality of life during chemotherapy.

Even in low-income contexts, simple interventions already show effect. In Ethiopia, the Healing Environments program by NGO MASS Design introduced basic alterations in community hospitals: natural light entry, cross ventilation, and soft colors. Results included improved patient recovery and increased satisfaction and lower turnover among health professionals: the environment is therapeutic for caregivers too.

A study published in the *International Journal of Environmental Research and Public Health* showed that inserting acoustic panels, plants, and local art in inpatient environments reduced stress markers by up to 28% in patients hospitalized for more than five days. This impact surpasses that of many first-line medications—without side effects. But this "environmental prescription" still does not appear in guidelines, much less in medical records.

Now, shall we talk about noise? Silence is one of modern medicine's most neglected therapies. Absence of noise allows vagal self-regulation, essential to reduce inflammation, modulate mood, and facilitate healing processes. In pediatric ICUs in the Netherlands, using headphones with nature sounds for premature babies reduced mechanical ventilation time and increased average daily weight gain. This is cutting-edge medicine ignored by biomedical orthodoxy.

Studies in US hospitals showed that high noise levels in ICUs are associated with increased blood pressure, heart rate, and cortisol levels in critical patients, which can be decisive in recovering bodies in fragile states needing a base to strengthen their immune system. In Brazil, research conducted at a university hospital in São Paulo revealed that continuous exposure to sounds above 60dB in hospital environments prolongs length of stay and increases delirium incidence in elderly patients. There's more: a systematic review published in the *Journal of Intensive Care* highlighted that interventions to reduce environmental noise, such as acoustic panels and staff awareness protocols, bring significant improvement in patient sleep quality, a crucial factor for cellular regeneration and immune recovery.

It borders on surrealism and invisibly surpasses professional ethics that hospital procedures often sacrifice patients' sleep for the convenience of professionals' schedules or that sunbathing is not offered as part of the infamous procedures. This negligence is still institutionally accepted, just as smoking inside a plane was accepted a few decades ago.

The same goes for smell. Hospital aromatherapy studies show that lavender and rosemary, in continuous diffusion, reduce preoperative anxiety and improve sleep in post-surgical patients. A hospital in Osaka, Japan, introduced this approach in oncology wards and reported a 23% reduction in severe insomnia episodes. Why, then, does anamnesis ignore smell, architecture ignore senses, and care ignore the body with senses interfering in health, treating all this as "superstitions" or "very alternative things"? It is interesting to note how initiatives activating smell are often understood as esoteric, or even childish, by people unaware of the neurochemical complexity behind olfactory interactions with the brain and body.

But the answer perhaps lies in the reductionist model still organizing care as a sum of exams, diagnoses, and standardized conducts. Everything escaping the measurable is treated as superfluous. But, we already spoke of this: this is a tool limitation, not reality. The body responds to where it is and alters all chemical dynamics forcefully.

Negligence of the physical surrounding is even graver when considering that the hospitalized patient is often in a state of perceptual hypersensitivity. Absence of control over light, noise, temperature, and privacy is, in itself, a stress vector. Karolinska Institutet researchers demonstrated that patients who could control room lighting and noise presented lower cortisol levels and fewer episodes of mental confusion. But this autonomy is systematically withdrawn, as if it were an accessory.

Emergency units are a case apart: they seem designed to increase the feeling of discomfort and coldness. Overcrowding, constant fluorescent lighting, absence of windows, alarms coming from unknown sources, and fragmented interaction with professionals create an environment resembling a process factory more than a care space. A multicenter study conducted in Latin America by PAHO/WHO showed that 72% of patients reported feelings of depersonalization during ER admissions, many describing the place as "freezing," "chaotic," or "violent to the senses." We don't even realize it; it's as if it had to be this way.

Many professionals still associate environmental comfort with luxury, as if caring for the surrounding were a sign of waste or ostentation. This belief is fed by decades of technical training separating the physical body from lived experience. But this dualism does not hold up against evidence: pain is amplified by negative environmental stimuli. Patients exposed to constant noise and intense brightness report pain levels up to 40% higher, even with the same analgesia. This is physiology, not fussiness.

In public units, the situation worsens. Inequality between public and private health units is brutal: public network patients often face deteriorated, poorly lit environments, with leaks, noise, bad smells, no ventilation. This is iatrogenic. Physical environmental precariousness increases anxiety, reduces trust in the team, generates autonomic nervous system hyperactivation, and can compromise the immune system. What should heal re-enacts the structural violence the patient already lives outside.

On the other hand, health plans have been exploring ambience marketing without necessarily incorporating environmental intelligence. Rooms with comfortable armchairs and coffee and sandwiches are offered as a sign of care, but often hide the same noises, stressful flows, and unwelcoming environment. The aesthetic, isolated from sensory intelligence, is makeup. What is truly expected is an environment helping to breathe, silence, process pain, reorganize body dynamics.

WHY CARE ENVIRONMENTS REMAIN HOSTILE

Modern hospital architecture, it is worth remembering, was born of war —and remains, largely, with its soul intact. Throughout the 20th century, the hospital building model was strongly inspired by concepts of control, surveillance, and order, derived from military and prison environments. In the early days of medicine's institutionalization, hospitals were thought of as places of isolation, death containment, and chaos neutralization. This heritage materializes to this day in endless corridors, wings separated by function, standardized artificial lighting, and the predominance of functional linearity over care organicity.

This physical design expresses a view on what caring means. Bed arrangement, ward position relative to nursing stations, absence of natural elements or sensory modulators - everything contributes, ironically, to consolidating a hospital experience centered on protocol compliance, as if its highest goal were fulfilling the protocol. Architecture reinforces the distance between technical knowledge and the experience of illness. Hospitals continue, mostly, to be environments designed to discipline bodies, not to restore the bond with health. This logic, inherited from the 19th century and maintained by inertia, translates into cold materials, washable surfaces, absence of identity in rooms, and an almost choreographed effort to ensure efficiency at the expense of what makes sense for a debilitated body, including its healing process.

Here, we are being subtle. In more critical cases, this can indeed be the difference between life and death for a patient. Sleep that cannot regulate itself can strongly compromise an already fragile immune system and increase mortality in case of hospital infection - which, even in environments claiming to prioritize hygiene and sterilization, remains a great "phantom killer," with no signs of reversing this frightening trend completely perverting the meaning of being in a hospital.

The impact of this on patients is profound. Absence of silence, excess artificial light at night, constant noise from machines, alarms, voices (often speaking unnecessarily loud), and footsteps are registered by the brain as threat signals. Studies on hospital noise pollution, such as those conducted by WHO and the *Journal of Environmental Psychology*, show noise levels in ICUs frequently exceed 80 decibels—far above limits considered safe for physiological rest.

In a public hospital in São Paulo, research conducted in 2020 by USP's School of Public Health demonstrated that 72% of patients reported waking up at least four times per night during hospitalization due to noises, lights, or routine interventions. Architecture and protocol did not dialogue with the patient's cycle, but with the institution's machinery. This type of mismatch is the rule.

Containment logic is also cruel in sectors like pediatrics and palliative care. In pediatric hospitals, absence of playful stimuli, environment standardization, and physical separation from parents create an environment intensifying the child's fear and stress. Architecture was not thought for playing, calming, caring for the bond. In many cases, children's spaces are restricted to colorful murals in cold corridors. The proposal's content is the same—only the color changes. In palliative care, the last days of life, which could be surrounded by silence, beauty, human warmth, and comfort, often happen in a room visually identical to that of a patient being operated on in two days (or in the same room).

The same situation repeats in mental health services. Environments designed for physical containment and monitoring, with mirrors, doors with viewports, locked windows, and absence of healthy sensory stimuli end up aggravating psychic suffering. The idea that risk must be avoided at all costs generates spaces punishing rather than welcoming. Patients with emotional crises are locked in environments that, in many cases, violate any current notion of mental health care.

Aggressive environments produce aggressive responses. Restorative environments activate the parasympathetic nervous system, reduce cortisol release, stabilize blood pressure, and facilitate regeneration. This is consolidated knowledge in neuroarchitecture and environmental psychology studies. An article published in the *Health Environments Research & Design Journal* analyzed over 600 articles on hospital design and found robust evidence that elements like natural light, visual access to nature, noise control, and space personalization reduce length of stay, medication use, and infection rates.

In 2018, the National Health Service of England launched a pilot program where palliative patients could choose elements of the inpatient environment (lighting, sounds, temperature, artwork, aromas) to ensure greater comfort and well-being. The impact was direct: 29% reduction in sedative use and 37% increase in perception of dignity in the dying experience, according to family surveys.

THEMATIC FOCUS: HOSPITAL - PLACE OF HEALING OR MACHINE OF ILLNESS?

Cold and Intermittent Fluorescent Light

⚠ **Impact:** Stimulates sympathetic system, suppresses melatonin, reduces HRV.
◍ **Conditions affected:** Insomnia, chronic pain, delirium, headache.
— **Why it persists:** Cost and construction standardization.
⇢ **Viable alternative:** Natural light, warm lamps with circadian spectrum.

Constant Alarms and Medical Equipment Noise

⚠ **Impact:** Continuous trigger of hypervigilance and clinical anxiety.
◍ **Conditions affected:** Elevated pressure, oxidative stress, worsening sleep, and burnout.
— **Why it persists:** Maximum monitoring culture.
⇢ **Viable alternative:** Smart alarms, modulated sounds, visual panels.

Absence of Windows, Plants, Landscape

⚠ **Impact:** Reduces neural connectivity, worsens mood and resilience.
◍ **Conditions affected:** Slow healing, depression, disorientation.
— **Why it persists:** Functionalist design; lack of norm.
⇢ **Viable alternative:** Biophilic environments, clinical gardens, hanging vegetation.

Chemical Hospital Odor

⚠ **Impact:** Aversive olfactory stimulus → nausea, anxiety, traumatic memories.
◍ **Conditions affected:** Reduced appetite, headache, flashbacks.
— **Why it persists:** Non-sensory hygienism.
⇢ **Viable alternative:** Clinical aromatherapy, organic odor neutralization.

Visual Uniformity (White Walls, Vinyl Floor, Absence of Symbology)

⚠ **Impact:** Disorients, suppresses affection and identity; aestheticizes alienation.
◍ **Conditions affected:** Depersonalization, anxiety, confusion in elderly.
— **Why it persists:** Economy and fear of "emotional excess."
⇢ **Viable alternative:** Architectural chromotherapy, contextual art, natural colors.

Barriers to Companion Presence

⚠ **Impact:** Interrupts affective safety and emotional co-regulation.
◍ **Conditions affected:** Delusions, emotional lability (intense and disproportionate mood changes), therapeutic dropout.
— **Why it persists:** Institutional fear of interference.
⇢ **Viable alternative:** Hospitals with full companionship, co-habitation protocols.

Absence of Visible Time (No Clocks, No Windows, No Ritual)

⚠ **Impact:** Deregulates circadian cycle, scrambles chronotypes, aggravates delusions.

◍ **Conditions affected:** Sleep disorders, nocturnal agitation, existential anguish.
— **Why it persists:** Invisibility of time in medical logic.
⇢ **Viable alternative:** Environments with natural time marking, chronobiological light.

Technical and Uncomfortable Furniture (Cold Chairs, Non-Ergonomic Beds)

⚠ **Impact:** Amplifies pain, prevents relaxation, compromises feeling of welcome.
◍ **Conditions affected:** Muscle pain, worsening of rheumatological and post-operative conditions, difficulty relaxing.
— **Why it persists:** Project focused on sterile functionality.
⇢ **Viable alternative:** Ergonomic armchairs, beds with warm textures, natural materials.

Impersonal Clinical Attire (Uniforms, Lab Coats, Touch Barriers)

⚠ **Impact:** Reinforces hierarchical distance and impersonality.
◍ **Conditions affected:** Fear, retraction, patient silence.
— **Why it persists:** Biomedical culture of visual authority.
⇢ **Viable alternative:** Humanized functional clothing, identification with name and role, colored clothes.

When we realize the environment, as built, frontally contradicts its objective (of healing), it becomes easier to understand the crisis the world lives in health and worrying data on complications or even deaths happening in hospitals due to factors different from the original disease motivating admission. It is not rare for patients admitted with a condition to pass away from a cause totally unrelated to the admission reason: it is the already fragile body being exposed to a battery of challenges imposed by an environment that does not care about what actually favors healing, or worse, with what can little by little totally undermine recovery chances.

INSTITUTIONALIZED HORROR: WHEN THE DOCTOR'S AGENDA IS MORE IMPORTANT THAN THE PATIENT'S LIFE

The logic of the medical agenda overriding patient sleep is a perfect portrait of care axis displacement in hospital environments. Waking a patient at 4 AM to collect blood, not because the exam needs to be done at this time, but because the doctor will make their 3-minute visit at 7 AM, reveals the institution organizes around professional availability, not clinical necessity.

And this pattern is omnipresent in various hospitals and rehabilitation centers inside and outside Brazil. A study conducted by Harvard Medical School in partnership with Brigham and Women's Hospital evaluated 93,000 admissions and found 45% of nocturnal lab tests had no clinical justification. Institutional agenda, not patient body, dictated routine. The consequence: sleep disorders, irritability, healing difficulty, immune system compromise, and everything cascading from there (the list is long and categorically represents life risk in more fragile bodies).

Similar episodes occur in medication administration, with standardized times for the team, without considering organism rhythm. Corticosteroids offered at night, contradicting morning administration recommendation. Diuretics given at day's end, compromising sleep. Exams requiring fasting requested out of standard, demanding unnecessary deprivations. All due to lack of articulation between care and institutional flow.

The result is what we can call "clinical iatrogenesis environments." Places operating on logic different from care physiology and causing health damage. These are institutions promoting ostensive but not restorative care; technical but not effective; continuous but not human (a function often falling on nursing professionals or psychologists, depending solely on goodwill of collaborators often also exhausted). The body does not sicken only from disease, but from how it is treated during disease.

This logic also reaches "waiting" spaces, which in many hospitals and clinics are true sensory deserts. Cold rooms, uncomfortable chairs, fluorescent lighting, TV on random channel, and absence of comforting stimuli reinforce alert and helplessness states. We are not talking merely of aesthetic discomfort, but a condition elevating stress levels, known to be linked to worse clinical outcomes. Neuroscience studies show impersonal environments activate the cerebral amygdala, region associated with vigilance and fear, sabotaging effects of medical interventions coming after.

The myopic premise of absolute functionality also imposes limits on patient intimacy, rest, and autonomy. By not permitting individuals to minimally personalize their space (with personal objects, photos, aromas, or small adaptations), the hospital reinforces the feeling of being system property, not protagonist of own healing process. This erasure is especially grave in longer admissions, like oncology or neurological rehabilitation, where environment ceases to be a transit place.

There is a type of violence or protocol negligence in how spaces impose themselves, unintended but continuous, and absence of a culprit with name and surname does not relieve suffering. It manifests in inability to close a curtain, absence of comfortable seating for family, standardized lighting invading face at night, uninterrupted sound of beeps and alarms. It is invisible, minimized, institutionalized violence sustained by safety and logistics arguments, but silently undermining well-being of those supposed to be in recovery process.

Hospitals daring to break this logic have reaped expressive results. Næstved Health Center in Denmark, designed by renowned architects for patients with complex health needs, replaced traditional hospital ambience with welcoming environments with community kitchens, accessible gardens, reading rooms, and living spaces. Clinical metrics improved: lower opioid consumption, higher treatment adherence, and better sleep quality.

Brazil also has incipient cases. Hospital Israelita Albert Einstein in São Paulo included in some units rooms with luminosity control, aromatherapy, soundtracks, and biophilic design—especially in palliative care. Hospital das Clínicas of USP Medical School, in partnership with Institute of Psychiatry, implemented sensory architecture project for psychiatric inpatient environments, with promising results in reducing agitation episodes.

PROTOCOLS AFFECTING SENSES — AND HEALTH

Medicine, historically, had in touch one of its first and most powerful diagnostic and therapeutic tools. The hand auscultating, holding, welcoming, was as essential as clinical gaze. But with technology advance, safety protocol hypertrophy, and institutionalized fear of error, touch was delegitimized, neutralized, converted into risk. Instead of proximity, it came to mean exposure. Instead of bond, it came to mean legal threat. This inversion corroded doctor-patient relationship and also an essential sensory dimension of care.

This phenomenon worsened with COVID-19 pandemic, normalizing physical distancing as protection. Masks, gloves, acrylic barriers, distancing protocols, all necessary in emergency context, were internalized. Professionals reported losing ability to recognize expressions, voice tones, subtle discomfort or emotion signs, because other's body became inaccessible. But problem predates pandemic. Since before, hospital environment was already hostile to sensory experience as whole.

A study conducted by Cleveland Clinic (2019) showed patients exposed to therapeutic soundtracks in controlled environment had 30% less need for painkillers in immediate post-op. Same study associated presence of natural aromas, like lavender and peppermint, to faster recovery in chronic pain patients. In Japan, *shinrin-yoku* practice, or "forest bathing," is already applied in internal clinical environments with real plants and natural shading, bringing expressive results in anxiety, blood pressure, and respiratory rate.

It is important to understand this is physiology. Vagus nerve activation, responsible for parasympathetic system and regulation of processes like digestion, heartbeats, and immune response, is directly influenced by tactile, auditory, and olfactory stimuli. Sensoriality is access route to vagal tone. And vagal tone is clinical proxy for well-being and physiological resilience.

This knowledge is not incorporated into practice and is curiously little discussed. In many hospitals, excess stimuli became part of problem: sound became aggression, light oppression, touch threat, time prison. In this scenario, body sickens more—or recovers less. Sensory architecture of healing was replaced by "aseptic" ambience ironically not avoiding mass hospital infections and continuous deaths by "hospital infection."

This disconnection between routine and physiological rhythm has practical consequences. Study published in *Journal of Clinical Sleep Medicine* (2019) demonstrated patients exposed to frequent sleep disturbances, like dawn blood collections, presented greater immune dysfunction and prolonged hospitalization time. In other words, it sickens. In American university hospital, after changing exam routine to more physiological times, there was 25% reduction in need for medication interventions for pain and anxiety.

In Japan, pediatric hospital in Saitama implemented, with local university support, program called *Kimochi no Shikumi*—something like "design of emotions." Wards were redesigned based on children's olfactory and tactile perception, with scented tracing paper partitions, soft fabrics, and use of natural materials. Children's stress rate during procedures fell 35% in three months, and engagement with professionals increased significantly.

In Brazil, initiatives exploring this depth are still rare, but some signal possible paths. Hospital Sírio-Libanês in São Paulo started pilot project some years ago in one of its ICUs using essential oil diffusers and playlists based on tone scales for calm induction. Reports show less nocturnal agitation and lower benzodiazepine need. Approach is still timid but demonstrates institutional openness.

In Canada, public hospitals began incorporating "sensory decompression room" for health professionals: 15-minute pause environments with binaural sound (stereo sound acting on mood regulation), amber lighting, aromatherapy, and chairs with gentle tactile stimulus. Program implemented during pandemic and, according to official report, resulted in 40% drop in burnout leaves in following quarter. Here, sensory is not just care instrument for patient, but for caregiver.

Important to highlight these are clinical interventions, based on neurophysiology and evidence, recognizing human body totality as care interface. Well-applied touch can reduce norepinephrine levels. Adequate music can modulate heart rate. Aroma can activate limbic system. Silent space can restore sleep and favor immune system. What these initiatives have in common is rupture with dehumanizing protocol. It is not about "improving ambience," but favoring healing where there was not, amazingly, a look for this.

There are also pilot projects investigating use of touch as expanded diagnostic tool. In palliative care centers in Germany, professionals are trained to recognize muscle tension patterns, skin texture, and micro-retractions as early pain signs, even in patients unable to verbalize. Response to this tactile listening has been anticipation of interventions and greater family adherence to team. In same line, University of Zurich studying impact of "silent tactile presence," simple continuous physical contact, without speech or additional stimulus, in advanced Alzheimer patients. Longitudinal study showed this type of presence stabilizes respiratory rate and reduces agitation episodes, and is deeply effective and little explored form of sensory care.

What is sought now with technology and research was, for long time, intuitive and organic in care craft. Nurses, midwives, family doctors knew power of room smell, hand temperature, environment music. But advance of technical-bureaucratic rationality, although bringing undeniable gains, dehydrated care until leaving it odorless, colorless, and tasteless - in best hypothesis. Recovering sensory is recovering human dimension of clinic, with intelligence and rigor.

CARE DESIGN AS STRATEGIC AXIS: ARCHITECTURE, PROTOCOLS, AND TECHNOLOGY

In many hospitals, inpatient experience is fragmented by systems not talking to each other: exam scheduling depends on one sector, internal transport on another, medication prescription on third, and discharge release on fourth department. Rule is these systems built from administrative sector logic. With this, small coordination failures generate delays, exam repetitions, forgetting essential steps, and chronic insecurity feeling.

Again: care design is not neutral. How spaces are built, systems designed, flows organized—all communicates intention and focus. Even if many leaders of these institutions (and perhaps because of it) treat these deficiencies as normal and out of reach, they are ones who can influence suppliers, developers, and partner companies. And if care environments more worried about counting procedures than cultivating health, then we face system having lost sight of its purpose.

Absence of listening spaces is also direct reflection of this institutional design. Offices with doors ajar, no acoustic isolation, attendance rooms with constant people circulation, absence of comfortable armchairs for companions or tables favoring horizontal dialogue between doctor and patient: all communicates, even involuntarily, listening is not priority. In survey by Institute for Patient and Family-Centered Care, patients experiencing environments with privacy and comfort described stronger bonds, better understanding of clinical picture, and greater treatment adherence.

Use of digital technologies in scheduling and initial triage also reveals how care can be shaped more by operational efficiency than encounter quality. Scheduling systems prioritizing 15-minute slots, even for complex cases, algorithms distributing patients by specialty without considering preferences, previous history, or emotional bond: all elements part of care ecosystem fragmenting experience and reducing human being to demand to be met, without commitment to outcome - which in our context affects "only" entire lives, or even interruption of life. And that is why, dear reader, space lacks in this work to "relieve" weight of all this uncomfortable normalized reality we live in - even with so much opportunity and proof of better paths.

Patient internal transport usually chapter apart in care disorganization. Long, little humanized routes, sometimes without adequate accompaniment, on uncomfortable stretchers, exposed to intense lighting and operational corridor noise. Movement within hospital should be seen as part of clinical journey, with potential to generate anxiety, pain, fear, and demand attention, listening, and welcoming.

And food? What can we say about it? Even if not case for many excellent private hospitals, hospital food often standardized, industrialized, served at fixed times not respecting appetite or patient metabolic condition, also shows how institutional design can sabotage recovery process. Absence of individualized look for food preferences, cultural restrictions, or emotional states related to food reduces nutrition to protocol, not integral therapeutic component.

Even furniture reveals institutional choices. Automated but uncomfortable beds. Companion chairs almost preventing prolonged stay.

Absence of balconies, small windows, opaque curtains preventing natural light entry. All interferes directly in circadian cycle regulation, time perception, and patient emotional recovery.

Care design needs to become strategic, transversal, and conscious health axis. Therefore, proposal to reconfigure health institutional design demands more than aesthetic reforms or logistical adjustments. Requires treating environment as co-therapist, clinical agent capable of amplifying care or silencing it. Studies from diverse institutions and relevant researchers prove well-planned environments reduce length of stay, decrease infections, and increase treatment adherence. Healing environment is not one just avoiding risks, it is one awakening feeling of safety, presence, recognition, and dignity.

This is leap we need to take. And this means integrating architects, engineers, designers, UX specialists, health professionals, and patients in collaborative processes from conception of any physical or digital structure. Care begins in project.

THEMATIC FOCUS: FACTORS FAVORING PATIENT HEALTH IN HOSPITAL ENVIRONMENTS

Natural Lighting

Impact: Presence of sunlight aids circadian rhythm regulation and improves mood.

Adequate Artificial Lighting

Impact: Lights with appropriate color temperature reduce visual fatigue and improve comfort.

Controlled Noise Levels

Impact: Silent environments promote rest and reduce stress.

Air Quality and Ventilation

Impact: Clean, well-ventilated air prevents respiratory infections.

Adequate Ambient Temperature

Impact: Comfortable temperatures avoid thermal discomfort and clinical complications.

Controlled Relative Humidity

Impact: Ideal humidity levels prevent mold and bacteria growth.

Efficient Ventilation

Impact: Adequate air renewal reduces pathogen concentration.

Presence of Windows

Impact: Access to external view improves psychological well-being.

Adequate Physical Space

Impact: Spacious environments avoid confinement feeling and facilitate mobility.

Acoustic Privacy

Impact: Sound isolation between environments guarantees confidentiality, security feeling, and comfort.

Soft Wall Colors

Impact: Soft tones promote relaxation and reduce anxiety.

Ergonomic Furniture

Impact: Comfortable, adapted furniture reduces injury risk and increases comfort.

Presence or View of Green Areas

Impact: Contact with nature accelerates recovery and reduces stress.

Clear Signage

Impact: Effective visual guidance reduces disorientation and anxiety.

Accessibility

Impact: Adapted environments guarantee safety and autonomy for all patients.

Odor Control

Impact: Environments with pleasant odors improve patient experience.

Reduction of Excessive Stimulus

Impact: Environments with controlled stimuli avoid sensory overload.

Spaces for Companions

Impact: Adequate areas for companions promote emotional support to patient.

Comfortable Waiting Areas

Impact: Pleasant waiting rooms reduce pre-attendance anxiety.

Presence of Ambient Music

Impact: Soft music can decrease pain perception and anxiety.

Adjustable Lighting

Impact: Allowing lighting adjustment offers patient control over environment.

Socialization Spaces

Impact: Common areas encourage interactions and reduce isolation.

Intuitive Layout

Impact: Logical design facilitates navigation and reduces confusion.

Personalized Spaces

Impact: Allowing patients to personalize space increases comfort.

Friendly Technology

Impact: Easy-to-use equipment reduces stress and increases autonomy.

Reduction of Unnecessary Alarms

Impact: Minimizing alarms avoids stress and auditory fatigue.

Meditation or Prayer Spaces

Impact: Areas dedicated to spiritual promote emotional well-being and influence immune system modulation.

Rigid Infection Control

Impact: Clean environments and effective protocols (mainly with collaborators, often transmission agents) prevent severe infections and contaminations.

Respected Circadian Rhythm

Impact: Environments respecting natural light cycles reduce delirium and insomnia.

Absence of Aggressive Hospital Odors

Impact: Reduction of nausea, anxiety, and discomfort in sensitive patients.

Natural Textures in Furniture and Walls

Impact: Materials like wood and stone increase welcoming feeling and trigger proven beneficial effects.

Nature Sounds as Sound Ambience

Impact: Environments with natural sounds reduce heartbeats and cortisol.

Presence of Pets or Animal-Assisted Therapies

Impact: Emotional improvement, stress reduction, and more stable vital signs.

Personalized Temperature

Impact: Individualized thermal control increases comfort and treatment adherence.

Absence of Direct Fluorescent Lighting

Impact: Diffused lighting reduces headaches and visual discomfort.

Local Cultural Elements in Environment

Impact: Environments reflecting patient culture promote psychological safety.

Possibility of Environment Control by Patient

Impact: Accessible light, sound, and bed buttons increase sense of autonomy and decrease stress.

Materials with Efficient Acoustic Absorption

Impact: Acoustic ceilings and panels reduce hospital noise.

Clinical Aromatherapy with Safe Essential Oils

Impact: Lavender and mint reduce nausea, anxiety, and pain. Diverse other plants and olfactory patterns studied and used for diverse beneficial effects.

Surfaces Pleasant to Touch

Impact: Cold metal surfaces increase feeling of discomfort and fear.

Presence of Interactive Artistic Elements

Impact: Interaction with art improves engagement and reduces feeling of imprisonment.

CHAPTER 11
CHRONIC DISEASES AND THE FAILURE OF THE FIX-IT MODEL

THE ACUTE LOGIC FACING THE CHRONIC CHALLENGE

Medicine was shaped by acute and interventional paradigms, and today it is visibly uncomfortable facing the chronic challenge. The tools that built extraordinary advances in treating infections, traumas, and emergencies systematically fail to offer sustainable answers to long-duration diseases. These conditions are slower, more silent, and more complex, traversed by social, emotional, and environmental factors challenging the linearity of conduct limited to prescriptions and exams. And at the center of this inadequacy is a structural error: treating chronic diseases as if they were infections. Instead of considering the progressive and multifactorial complexity of these conditions, the corrective model persists in operating through isolated episodes, focusing on remediating biomarkers or visible symptoms.

From the patient's point of view, this approach has a high cost. Not only in the financial sense but in the sense of the absence of meaning. An individual living with chronic pain, fatigue, metabolic oscillations, or recurrent emotional suffering who is nevertheless considered "stable" by their routine exams experiences a violent mismatch between their experience and what is validated by medicine. This dissonance has a name: clinical invalidation.

Even in health systems with visible efforts to be more integrated, like the SUS in Brazil or the NHS in the UK, the fragmentation between primary, specialized, and hospital care is an open wound, especially in chronic patient care. Everything we have already addressed here gains weight: the lack of interoperability between systems, the duplication of exams, the absence of unified medical records, and the ignorance of the patient's integral history turn the clinical path into a labyrinth, not a care journey.

For decades, we have accumulated solid evidence that success in controlling chronic diseases requires continuity, bonding, listening, adaptation, and daily support. The DAWN study (Diabetes Attitudes, Wishes and Needs), conducted in 13 countries with more than 5,000 people with diabetes, revealed that psychosocial factors are as determinant for glycemic control as biomarkers. Yet, clinical practice continues to prioritize laboratory metrics while ignoring despair, loneliness, fear of complications, or the shame of failing to follow the recommended diet —even though the literature is clear on the subject.

This is why the dichotomy between knowing and doing the best for the patient worsens so much in the field of chronic diseases. It is not a lack of guidelines: there are robust management guidelines for diabetes, hypertension, dyslipidemia, asthma, obesity, etc. But these documents were created based on population evidence, not individual realities. When mechanically transposed to the clinic, they fail to recognize that the patient is a social, affective organism with habits, routines, and concrete limitations. The guideline recommending walking 30 minutes a day makes no sense for the patient living in a violent community, without sidewalks, and without even free time in the day to walk.

Adherence—that concept as talked about as it is misunderstood, which we will treat in depth in another volume—is treated, in corrective logic, as a moral virtue of the patient, not as a relational construction. They are expected to obey even when recommendations conflict with their routine, culture, language, and suffering, as if "wanting" were enough to succeed. This reasoning, besides being outdated, is cruel: it ignores social determinants, cognitive barriers, health illiteracy, traumas, anguish, and the very fatigue chronic illness imposes.

The case of obesity is classic: it is a multifactorial condition with genetic, psychological, social, economic, and environmental roots. But it is still treated mostly through the prism of willpower and moral deficit. Correction is directed at the body, through diets, medications, surgeries, while the context sustaining weight gain, when it appears, is peripheral. Just as with the diabetic patient who is instructed to "have discipline" but lives anxiously and surrounded by ultra-processed foods, animal fat (linked to type 2 diabetes development), aggressive advertising, and lack of community support.

These evidences are still treated as "alternative," while the less effective model remains hegemonic, even being known to be ineffective. But why? The corrective model is simple to measure, profitable for fee-for-service remuneration, and easily replicable by protocols. It generates administrative predictability and is, therefore, a convenient institutional solution, even if clinically insufficient. Breaking it requires more than technical knowledge: it requires changing culture, indicators, medical training, institutional architecture, and digital solutions. And it also requires making clear that not seeking the best for the patient flirts with a lack of professional ethics.

Remote monitoring programs via digital health solutions, in theory, should serve to support patients, anticipate decompensations, and modulate conduct based on continuous data. But in many cases, they are used as mere alert sensors: the device registers the problem and generates an automatic response, without space for listening or personalization. Digitized correction remains correction, only faster.

Behind the scenes of clinical routine, doctors confess among colleagues that they no longer know what to say to the diabetic patient who, year after year, cannot control their blood sugar. Nurses report feeling guilty for not being able to truly help the patient with chronic obstructive pulmonary disease quit smoking. Psychologists realize that the anxious conditions they treat are deeply linked to food insecurity, unresolved traumas, and lack of life purpose. And all these professionals, when operating under corrective logic, feel powerless; they know something is missing.

The point is that this perception of limit needs to be seen as a turning point. The exhaustion of the corrective model, when assumed with intellectual honesty, opens space for a new architecture of care: broader, more connected, more adaptive.

THEMATIC FOCUS: RIGHT TOOLS IN THE WRONG PLACE - WHY ACUTE MEDICINE DOES NOT SUIT THE CHRONIC CHALLENGE

Conduct Based on Rigid Protocols and Guidelines

- **Historical Origin:** War and field medicine (NATO, post-war WHO).
- **Original Function:** Standardize decisions in imminent risk situations.
- **Chronic Context:** Ignores individual variations, biopsychosocial context, and does not respond to longitudinal complexity.
- **Necessary Transition:** Adaptive protocols, built based on journey and continuous clinical dialogue.

Removal of Causal Agent (Virus, Bacteria, Physical Trauma)

- **Historical Origin:** 19th-century infectious medicine.
- **Original Function:** Rapidly eliminate the cause to restore homeostasis.
- **Chronic Context:** Chronic diseases do not have a "single agent"—they have multiple interdependent vectors.
- **Necessary Transition in Care:** Causal network reasoning, with functional and systemic mapping.

Resolution by Spot Medication or Surgical Procedure

- **Historical Origin:** 20th-century technological advance, pharmaceutical and surgical boom.

- **Original Function:** Rapid interventions for functional return.
- **Chronic Context:** Generates control palliatives, drug dependence, and medicalization without restructuring.
- **Necessary Transition:** Integrated multiple interventions, with patient protagonism.

Symptom Control as Clinical End

- **Historical Origin:** Clinical emergencies: pain, fever, hypertensive crisis, trauma.
- **Original Function:** Avoid immediate suffering or death.
- **Chronic Context:** Chronifies conditions by not acting on slow and silent causes.
- **Necessary Transition:** Continuous monitoring focused on function, vitality, and trajectory reversal.

Medical Discharge as Sign of Success

- **Historical Origin:** Bed turnover logic and hospital efficiency.
- **Original Function:** Release the patient after resolved acute event.
- **Chronic Context:** Chronic patient has relapses, fluctuations, and needs sustained bonds.
- **Necessary Transition:** Longitudinal care models, with coordination and relational continuity.

Vertical Specialization of Care (Cardiologist, Nephrologist, etc.)

- **Historical Origin:** Expansion of post-Flexnerian biomedical knowledge, mechanistic and disease-focused.
- **Original Function:** Deepen experience on specific body systems.

- **Chronic Context:** Fragments care, disconnects knowledges, and prevents whole view.
- **Necessary Transition:** Articulated multiprofessional teams with horizontal and integrative vision.

Laboratory Exams as Main Decision Criterion

- **Historical Origin:** 20th-century laboratory medicine.
- **Original Function:** Confirm or exclude hypothesis based on objective biomarkers.
- **Chronic Context:** Chronic diseases are functional, fluctuating, contextual—often without clear "laboratory alteration."
- **Necessary Transition:** Integration of markers with listening, narrative, and contextual data.

Short, Productivist, Demand-Oriented Clinical Time

- **Historical Origin:** Massive hospital and outpatient culture.
- **Original Function:** Attend high volume with acute resoluteness.
- **Chronic Context:** The chronic demands time, listening, bond reconstruction, and behavioral change.
- **Necessary Transition:** Longer consultations, agreed care plans, and evolutionary listening.

MODERN MEDICINE FAILED BY USING ITS BEST TOOLS ON THE WRONG TARGETS. CHRONIC DISEASES DO NOT NEED A SPOT ATTACK, BUT A RECONSTRUCTION ECOSYSTEM. AS LONG AS CARE REMAINS FORMATTED BY ACUTE LOGIC, THE RESULT WILL CONTINUE TO BE A CYCLE OF RELAPSES, CLINICAL DEPENDENCE, SILENT FRUSTRATION OF ALL INVOLVED, AND OVERLOADED SYSTEMS.

THE CLINICAL FRAGMENTATION THAT SABOTAGES CONTINUITY

The SUS has faced this challenge with the Family Health Strategy, integrating teams composed of family and community doctors, nurses, community health agents, and other professionals. These teams act coordinately to offer continuous and comprehensive care, especially for patients with chronic conditions and vulnerable populations. The *Melhor em Casa* (Better at Home) program, aimed at home care, also brings important learnings. Still limited in scale, the model shows how multidisciplinary teams, when well-articulated, manage to offer continuous care, more humane and less hospital-centric. The challenge now is to expand, qualify, and integrate this experience into primary care networks, with technology and management centered on the patient cycle.

When we look at integrated care models that have advanced most in chronic disease care, such as the *Chronic Care Model*, developed by the MacColl Center in the United States, we perceive a common point: the reorganization of care around the patient's time. This includes everything from support between consultations (asynchronous communication, symptom triage, automated alerts) to the articulation of multiple professionals around a flexible therapeutic plan. Implementation of this model showed significant improvement in control indicators for diabetes, asthma, depression, and hypertension.

Brazil, even with great structural inequalities, possesses some inspiring experiences pointing in this direction. The Home Care Program of the Municipal Health Secretariat of Belo Horizonte implemented multiprofessional teams with therapeutic plans built together with the patient and their family. Studies conducted by the municipal management itself pointed to a good reduction in readmissions and improvement in quality of life reported by patients with chronic conditions like COPD, heart failure, and diabetes. What sustains these results is how technology is inserted into a care network.

A study conducted in 17 countries showed that more than 60% of patients with type 2 diabetes feel their health professionals do not understand the emotional challenges associated with the disease. And this gap directly impacts treatment adherence. It is not about offering psychotherapy sessions at every consultation (as skeptics might ironically suggest), but about incorporating a more attentive look at context, invisible suffering, hesitations shaping clinical behavior, and feasible strategies for more forceful influence on the root cause.

In the field of digital technologies, we have promising advances. Remote monitoring platforms, wearable devices with predictive alerts, risk algorithms adjusted to clinical trajectory—all this already exists. Recent studies have demonstrated that using AI platforms for symptom triage in patients with chronic diseases can considerably reduce response time to acute events, provided it is integrated with clinical listening and human validation. What works is the combination of presence, prediction, and personalization.

A patient with diabetes can have their blood sugar decompensated for weeks without anyone noticing, not for lack of data, but for lack of an architecture connecting this data to the patient's clinical biography.

From the moment it is recognized that emotional suffering is not a "side effect" of the disease, but an integral part of the chronic experience, care reorganizes. Studies with HIV patients show that including continuous psychosocial support in the therapeutic plan also improves immunological indicators. In regions where the system is most overloaded, this inadequacy becomes institutionalized negligence.

70% of public health system resources in the UK are destined for patients with chronic conditions, but less than 20% of care strategies are designed for continuity. The rest of the budget flows to crisis containment, avoidable hospitalizations, complications that could have been prevented with closer monitoring. This mathematics of waste is perhaps the most scandalous statistic of contemporary health—and yet, one of the least discussed.

Data from the Institute of Supplemental Health Studies indicate that chronic patients account for 83% of hospital admissions in health plan operators in Brazil, and for more than 80% of care costs. Yet, the immense majority of chronic management programs boils down to sending generic messages and monitoring biometric parameters without context. The result is a theater of care, where the patient appears as a number, technology becomes makeup, and billing does very well, thank you.

Health innovation has been captured by a logic prioritizing scalability over depth. And this is lethal when we speak of chronicity and complex realities. Because what the chronic patient needs, often, is not a new monitoring app, but one that deepens and connects their condition with realistic and pragmatic actions, considering their individual needs and improving their quality of life. Here, the challenge of transdisciplinarity becomes evident.

There are exceptions, of course. The "patient-centered medical home" model, mentioned earlier, has variants in Canada, the Netherlands, and Australia successfully incorporating the concept of longitudinality. In the Netherlands, the "Buurtzorg" model reorganized home care based on small autonomous nursing teams accompanying the same patients over months or years.

This leads us to an unavoidable ethical point: the corrective model is inadequate in its time architecture. It operates from the premise that care can be compressed into clinical windows of a few minutes, between one computer screen and another, whereas chronic care demands extended presence and a dynamic different from that offered in the immense majority of cases. It demands space for the unspoken, for the unforeseen, for what only appears when returning to the same patient more than once—and in this meantime, which is where life (and health) happens. This is the intelligence of repetition and consistency.

The corrective model also fails to recognize the social environment's role as co-author of health or disease. A hypertensive patient living in a violent neighborhood, without access to fresh food, with precarious transport and exhausting work routines does not need an automatic reminder to take medicine, but a system understanding what conditions their body. The logic of isolated prescription, without articulation with intersectoral policies, ends up attributing to the individual a responsibility that, often, they cannot fulfill or, even fulfilling, will not be sufficient.

It is common for health professionals to need to "hunt" for information in different systems, call colleagues, check with the patient if a certain exam was done. This time lost searching for data is time missing to listen, examine, and think.

Even clinical protocols, which should guide with intelligence, often worsen fragmentation: a patient with hypertension, diabetes, and depression will be subjected to three distinct tracks, with goals, exams, and conducts that most likely do not converse with each other. The result is disconnected care, overloaded with tasks, without prioritization and without listening, as if the body were not something extremely complex and interconnected.

The Family Health Strategy, when well implemented, represents a bet on continuity. Teams accompanying families over time, knowing the territory, building bonds. But even this model faces challenges, such as professional turnover, demand overload, and support system fragility. In the private sector, some health plans have invested in care coordination models: implementing "health navigators," remote monitoring platforms, and chronic management programs are important steps, but are still sporadic initiatives, often disconnected from primary care and without integration with other care levels.

CHAPTER 12
HEALTH AS A SYSTEM OF POTENCY

DECONSTRUCTING THE LOGIC OF ABSENCE

Modern medicine, in seeking to quantify and control health, has ended up restricting it to a limiting concept: absence of symptoms, absence of pain, absence of laboratory alterations. This minimalist definition, although operationally very useful for protocols, deeply impoverishes the human experience of "living well" and ignores the quantity of forces that sustain someone's health.

When something is defined by what it is not, its identity is shifted to negation. Defining health as "not being sick" is equivalent to defining joy as "not being sad": a dangerous simplification. The absence of disease does not guarantee the presence of vitality, creative energy, or disposition for a world that demands much—from the body and the mind.

Health is, first of all, the capacity to tolerate environmental variations. A healthy organism is one that can oscillate, reinvent itself, create new balances in the face of the unpredictable, and not just one that remains within a statistical reference range. This notion of adaptability, well-supported scientifically, contrasts with dominant medical thinking, which relies on Gaussian curves and standardized laboratory values to define "normality."

The negative definition of health is reinforced by the very structure of health services, which are almost always activated in the face of a symptom, a collapse, a cry for help—and are structured for this. It is not just the concept that is biased: it is the entire operational logic. Little is taught about cultivating vitality, preventing decline, or following the patient's functional curve based on their potentials, and this space is being intensely occupied by professionals called "alternative" and by social media, where countless profiles bring, often intuitively, information helping people seek this vitality. And it is interesting to observe that this information had little space where it would be expected, in health systems, where this same information has always been treated as secondary, off-script, irrelevant in a way.

The logic of "defect hunting" has been very well instrumentalized by the pharmaceutical industry, which over decades expanded the concept of disease to include asymptomatic conditions, or "pre-something." From pre-diabetes to pre-Alzheimer's, from osteopenia to borderline cholesterol, risk zones were created which, while potentially offering another opportunity to act on reversal, end up justifying early chemical interventions, even when there is no suffering or functional loss—and neither forceful nor preventive actions. As a warning, epidemiologist John Ioannidis says we live today in an "epidemic of diagnoses" that does not necessarily improve people's health.

Language itself reflects this conceptual imprisonment. When one says someone "recovered their health," it is presupposed that it is something one has or does not have, like an object. This reinforces the idea that health is a static state, which can be lost and then found again. It happens that health is a continuous process, a dynamic balance among multiple factors in constant negotiation: genetic, environmental, emotional, social, spiritual.

This is exactly why many contemporary currents of psychology and integrative medicine have been proposing the concept of salutogenesis. The issue lies in the capacity to generate meaning, cohesion, life structure—elements escaping traditional clinical measurements.

Salutogenesis recognizes that health is not a fixed point, but a spectrum between two poles: the pathological and the healthy. We are all somewhere on this scale, oscillating all the time. What matters is the movement, the direction of the trajectory, and the resources we mobilize to move forward. This view is liberating because it takes the patient out of the position of "sick person waiting for a fix" and invites them to co-create their own health from the circumstances in which they live.

But many health professionals, trained in predominantly biomedical curricula, remain uncomfortable with the idea of dealing with emotional or existential aspects. Science, in its legitimate quest for precision, ended up building walls against everything that cannot be measured, even if due to technical limitations.

Seeing health as presence invites us to create new indicators capable of capturing well-being more sensitively. This does not mean abandoning traditional biomarkers, but complementing them with functional and relational measures, previously discarded as intangible, which technology already allows us to measure. We face a historic choice: continue operating under the logic of absence, or migrate to a new paradigm where health is recognized as a field of potency. This transition is not simple, but without it, we will continue treating bodies without caring for lives—and confusing biological silence with existential fullness.

Potency as a Vital Axis: Regeneration, Adaptation, and Meaning

Potency, when understood as a vital axis of health, shifts our gaze from correction to creation. A healthy organism is not one that only "functions within parameters," but one capable of responding to the world intelligently, variedly, and coherently with its own limits and desires. Potency is, ultimately, the art of not just surviving, but of continuing to become.

Biologically, this potency manifests clearly in regenerative processes accompanying us throughout life. Epithelial tissue constantly renews; the liver is capable of regenerating up to two-thirds of its mass after injury; bone marrow produces billions of new cells per day; new neural connections form all the time. In moments of wound or trauma, the body responds with a complex choreography of controlled inflammation, cellular recruitment, collagen reorganization, tissue closure, all without the need for a conscious command. Potency is inscribed in biology as a silent foundation. We even know now that experiencing adverse, frustrating situations, or those symbolizing a rupture, are capable of reorganizing and activating our brain in such a way that we can become "smarter" after the body's reaction to a frustration or difficult situation.

More than repairing, the organism learns from experience. Neuroplasticity studies show the adult brain continues creating new synaptic connections throughout life, especially when challenged by meaningful experiences. Recent research, such as Michael Merzenich's and Norman Doidge's group, reveals the nervous system is capable of reorganizing after trauma, strokes, and injuries, recovering functions considered lost.

Epigenetics reinforces this perspective by showing our genes operate as scores modulated by the environment. Stimuli like food, sleep, affective bond, physical activity, and emotional experiences have the power to activate or deactivate genes and modulate inflammatory, hormonal, and immunological processes. Moshe Szyf and Michael Meaney's work shows early maternal care experiences affect stress-related gene expression, with effects persisting throughout life.

Potency also manifests in the immunological sphere. The immune system is not just a defense force, but a conductor of internal balance, constantly negotiating with the environment. Recent research on the concept of "immunotolerance" shows a healthy organism is one knowing how to coexist with potentially aggressive agents without initiating destructive responses. The capacity to distinguish threat from noise is, in this sense, one of the most refined expressions of potency. A potent body is not one attacking everything; it is one knowing how to choose its battles. This concept appears clearly in studies on gut microbiota. The presence of billions of microorganisms in the digestive tract is not an anomaly, but an evolutionary alliance sustaining metabolic, neurological, and immunological processes. A healthy microbiome participates in neurotransmitter synthesis, HPA (hypothalamic-pituitary-adrenal) axis modulation, intestinal barrier protection. Microbial diversity is potency. Conversely, loss of this diversity, due to excessive antibiotic use, ultra-processed diet, chronic stress, reduces the body's adaptive capacity and paves the way for systemic imbalances.

Potency is also coherence between systems. Health is not the isolated good functioning of each organ, but the ensemble's capacity to maintain harmony even under pressure. The concept of homeodynamics, proposed by scientists like Ilya Prigogine and Stuart Kauffman, replaces the idea of static homeostasis with a vision of fluid balance, in constant negotiation. Healthy organisms maintain their parameters through plasticity, through flexibility in the face of external instabilities. It is this dynamic intelligence allowing response to stress factors.

A healthy subject is one who can feel sadness without sinking into it, who recognizes pain without identifying completely with it, who tolerates life's ambiguity without fleeing to rigid narratives. Potency, here, merges with the capacity to be present with wholeness before what is. In psychology, authors like Donald Winnicott and Carl Rogers pointed to this state as an essential condition of emotional maturation: not avoiding suffering, but having internal resources to traverse it.

A potent patient is not one who "has no symptoms," but one possessing internal tools, external networks, and repertoire to understand and deal with their symptoms. This implies recognizing the importance of culture, meaning, spirituality, art, the body in motion, intimacy. And, therefore, it requires care that is transdisciplinary and technically refined at the same time.

The **Blue Zones** are regions mapped by researcher Dan Buettner and a National Geographic team, where there is an unusual concentration of centenarians, with low prevalence of chronic diseases and high quality of life into advanced ages. Among them are Okinawa (Japan), Sardinia (Italy), Ikaria (Greece), Nicoya (Costa Rica), and Loma Linda (California). Despite cultural differences, these communities share common elements: a diet based on whole and local foods, strong social connections, clear life purpose, moderate and natural physical activity, adequate sleep, and a life rhythm respecting the body. Studies like this show that factors most strongly associated with a long and healthy life are not only genetic or nutritional, but relational and existential, and even if apparently trivial, maintain the organism in flow, silently regenerating each day. Potency, here, is rhythm, is lightness, is continuity.

And this notion appears in integrative therapeutic practices placing the body in intelligent movement: yoga, dance, active meditation, tai chi chuan. As studies on meditation show, like Lazar et al. (published in *Neuroreport* in 2005), breathing techniques and body awareness impact cortical thickness increase, particularly in brain regions linked to attention and sensory processing, suggesting meditation can compensate for age-related cortical thinning. Science begins mapping what ancient traditions already knew: health is not only in organs, but in how we move and relate to the world.

This vision is not spiritualist; it is systemic. Potency is the opposite of passivity, and manifests as much in metabolism as in cognition, joints, muscles, and bonds. When cultivated with attention, it can transform a functionally limited life into an existentially rich life. And when ignored, it transforms apparently functional bodies into lives chronically devoid of vitality, spiritless.

Potency is also revealed in the system's capacity to anticipate collapse. Instead of reacting when there is a failure, a potent organism is capable of perceiving small variations and correcting routes before damage sets in. This predictive intelligence is one of the most sophisticated characteristics of living systems, present from cellular physiology to complex daily decision-making. An adaptive system does not wait to break; it reorganizes preventively. And this should also apply to healthcare.

In the fields of affective neuroscience and behavioral psychology, there is decisive evidence that positive emotions, healthy bonds, and a sense of meaning are associated with better immunity, lower cardiovascular risk, and greater longevity. Barbara Fredrickson, in her broaden-and-build theory of positive emotions, shows how positive affective states, even the briefest, expand cognitive repertoires, reinforce social connections, and activate physiological recovery circuits.

This state of "organized vitality" requires minimal material conditions: housing, adequate food, restorative sleep, time for rest—but also recognition. Being seen, being heard, being validated in one's own life experience contributes to health. In marginalized communities, psychosocial support programs, qualified listening, and strengthening of bonds are often more effective than purely pharmacological interventions.

All this points to a possible and necessary redesign of care practices. Medicine, when updated with this view, ceases to be a field of repairs and becomes a field of cultivation, recognizing the body's natural regeneration processes, emotional adaptation circuits, experiential knowledges. A loss can reveal meaning, a symptom can be a relevant request for reorganization.

THEMATIC FOCUS: BODY POTENCY LEVELS BEFORE BREAKING

An illustrative functional transition showing the body's potency curve before collapse happens, the stages where medicine sees nothing, measures nothing, and does nothing—while the organism is already in adaptation, compensation, attempt, and warning mode. The proposal is to transform health into a non-binary potency continuum of vitality, with milestones the current system ignores but can be integrated by a "potency medicine."

Imagine a descending curve of potency → until total dysfunction. Traditional medicine only acts in the last third.

✦ Phase 1: Full Potency in Adaptation

🫀 What the body is doing: Compensates for micro-aggressions (irregular sleep, micro-inflammations, emotional tension) with neuroendocrine elasticity and immune modulation.
🩺 Traditional Medicine: "Perfect health" / "nothing to treat."
🔎 Ignored Signs: Subtle mood variations, drop in mental performance, mild digestive oscillations.
⇢ Potency-Oriented Medicine: Strengthen rhythm, self-awareness, variability, and emotional expression.

✦ Phase 2: Silent Balance Adjustments

🫀 What the body is doing: Changes basal pattern to maintain functionality: starts living "on reserves."
🩺 Traditional Medicine: "Normal exams" / "common tiredness."
🔎 Ignored Signs: Non-restorative sleep, irritability, stimulus dependence (caffeine, sugar), altered menstrual cycles.
⇢ Potency-Oriented Medicine: Measure vitality (HRV, sleep, bond, energy), intervene before rupture.

✦ Phase 3: Visible but Subclinical Compensation

🫀 What the body is doing: Starts expressing signs of overload: modulates symptoms to maintain survival.
🩺 Traditional Medicine: "Anxiety," "tension," "lifestyle."
🔎 Ignored Signs: Libido drop, binge eating, mild forgetfulness, diffuse pain.
⇢ Potency-Oriented Medicine: Listen to the body as functional expression and reorganize concrete life.

✦ Phase 4: Functional Pre-Damage

🫀 What the body is doing: Minimal physiological alterations appear, not yet crossing diagnostic thresholds.
🩺 Traditional Medicine: "Everything still fine in exams," "normal for age," "need to take care."
🔎 Ignored Signs: Pre-hypertension, altered blood sugar, low ferritin, mild dysbiosis.
⇢ Potency-Oriented Medicine: Reverse dysfunctional adaptive pattern with potency plan.

✦ Phase 5: Partial Clinical Rupture

🫀 What the body is doing: No longer sustains self-regulation—symptom becomes localized collapse.
🩺 Traditional Medicine: "Now we have something to treat."
🔎 Ignored Signs: Migraine, gastritis, insomnia, burnout, PCOS, prediabetes.
⇢ Potency-Oriented Medicine: Act on broad collapse vectors and effective solutions.

✦ Phase 6: Installed and Chronified Dysfunction

🫀 What the body is doing: Gives up modulating—enters clinical survival mode.

🩺 Traditional Medicine: Continuous corrective treatment.
🔎 Ignored Signs: Polypharmacy, loss of meaning, adherence without autonomy.
⇢ Potency-Oriented Medicine: Here, rebuild remains, with continuous and comprehensive look.

EVIDENCE SUSTAINING HEALTH AS POTENCY

The beauty of health as potency is that it manifests elegantly and forcefully in different contexts around the world. There are entire regions, specific populations, clinical programs, and care experiments already living, organically, this more affirmative logic of well-being. And most fascinating is that these experiences are rigorously observable.

These data gain even more relevance when confronted with alarming numbers from traditional corrective medicine: growing costs with chronic disease treatments, indiscriminate use of multiple medications, and mental health indicators continuing to deteriorate even in technologically advanced countries. The Blue Zones offer no miracles, but relevant clues to practices sustaining the body throughout life, at incomparably lower cost. This should sound an alarm in the current system, insisting on neglecting what clearly works.

Also revealing are evidences from disease reversal studies with lifestyle changes. Cardiologist Dean Ornish conducted research showing intensive lifestyle changes, such as whole-food plant-based diet, light exercise, meditation, and social support, can reverse coronary atherosclerosis progression. In an emblematic study, patients with severe heart disease demonstrated arterial plaque reduction, improved cardiac function, and expressive drop in hospitalization rates, all without surgery or high-dose medication.

These discoveries challenge the traditional concept placing chronic diseases as inevitable and irreversible conditions. What Ornish and other researchers showed is that the body has regeneration mechanisms that can be activated when the right elements are cultivated consistently. Also decisive is the work of Elizabeth Blackburn, Nobel laureate in Medicine, and her research partner Elissa Epel, demonstrating that practices like meditation, healthy eating, restorative sleep, and positive relationships are directly associated with telomere preservation (protective chromosome ends), whose integrity is linked to cellular aging. In other words, emotional states and daily habits have measurable impact on biological longevity. Living with vitality is not a metaphor; it is a molecular phenomenon. It is also interesting to observe how these approaches (highly effective in many cases) are systematically placed at healthcare margins, as less qualified, less scientific, or even less serious alternatives. Of course, efficacy evidence must be sought, and this is precisely our point: there are many. But as long as medicine remains hermetically isolated from other disciplines and advanced scientific knowledge (perhaps less pharmacological, but no less scientific), advancement will not stop. Other professions and specialties will continue emerging as a natural response to a clear market opportunity gap: that of healthcare with meaning, respecting body and life complexity.

These sophisticated discoveries only confirm something many traditional cultures always knew: health is not fragment, it is flow. Ayurvedic medicine, Traditional Chinese Medicine, ancestral integrative practices from the Americas and Africa recognized centuries ago the interdependence between body, mind, and environment. What was once considered empirical knowledge now begins to be validated in the laboratory, and there is no contradiction in this. On the contrary: the most refined contemporary science is rediscovering, with humility, much of what popular wisdom preserved.

In the mental health field, evidence also points to potency paths. Programs like **Open Dialogue**, developed in Finland, have revolutionized care for people in severe psychic distress by replacing the classic biomedical model with listening networks, open dialogue with family, and patient protagonism. Results are impressive: greater patient autonomy, lower antipsychotic medication use, fewer hospitalizations, and a recovery rate far superior to traditional models' average.

Even in oncology, where the war-against-cancer imaginary is dominant, more integrated approaches begin to emerge. Centers like MD Anderson Cancer Center have been incorporating complementary practices, such as acupuncture, nutritional therapy, psychological support, and body practices, as part of standard treatment, expanding it based on evidence that integral care improves adherence, reduces side effects, and contributes to patient general well-being, with direct impact on recovery trajectory.

It is also true that social determinants of health, such as education, income, access to quality food, safety, transport, and housing, account for a very considerable slice of health outcomes, more than medical services themselves. Studies from the Robert Wood Johnson Foundation and Centers for Disease Control and Prevention show only 10 to 20% of factors impacting health are directly linked to clinical care. The rest lies in how people live, work, sleep, relate, and eat.

And more recent technologies, like artificial intelligence, wearable sensors, and monitoring apps, have shown they can favor this dynamic when used to promote patient awareness and engagement.

All this evidence invites us to a posture change: instead of waiting for disease to manifest to act, we can build solutions, routines, relationships, and systems cultivating health before failure. Potency is not spontaneous, but cultivable. It is not born of chance, but of the conjunction between choices, conditions, bonds, and attention. And most importantly: this can be done sustainably, with lower cost and greater impact.

POTENCY AS FUTURE CLINICAL RESOURCE

It is curious and deeply revealing to realize how much potency, despite its evident presence in life phenomena, remains absent from conventional clinical practices. In the era of scientific advances and predictive technologies, health care still revolves mostly around what is broken, what can be fixed. This omission is structural, rooted in training still shaping most university curricula. In most medical and nursing schools, little is taught about identifying silent resilience, the emotional response insisting on manifesting despite diagnosis, and how all this connects and directly interferes in health.

Primary care physicians are often not trained to discuss sleep, sexuality, spirituality, or support networks with their patients. And these themes are, according to patients themselves, central to their health perception. There is a gap between what the patient experiences and what the doctor learned to see, and this gap costs dearly: in adherence, bond, therapeutic efficacy, and sustainable results over time.

Worse than ignoring potency is treating it as irrelevant. Many health professionals, lacking repertoire or under institutional pressure, discourage any patient initiative straying from the biomedical script. A woman deciding to walk every day to deal with her grief is seen as "doing what she can." A man finding respite from anxiety in tending an urban garden is praised as "resilient," but rarely is this incorporated as a formal clinical strategy. In both cases, what should be recognized as an active health nucleus is treated as a peripheral curiosity, which in more extreme contexts gets invalidated.

This hollowing of potency as a clinical resource also manifests in the absence of space for integrative practices in traditional protocols. Despite hundreds of studies proving benefits of meditation, mindfulness, conscious breathing, and acupuncture in diverse contexts, from chronic pain to anxiety, oncology to cardiovascular rehabilitation, these practices remain niche offerings. The National Center for Complementary and Integrative Health has gathered dozens of analyses showing statistically relevant efficacy of various integrative approaches.

The Southcentral Foundation in Alaska promoted a deep transformation in approach. Instead of considering people served merely as "patients," the foundation adopted the term "customer-owner." This concept reflects a fundamental change: individuals are active participants responsible for their own health decisions. The Nuka System of Care, created by the foundation itself, aims to build lasting bonds based on mutual trust, active listening, and co-responsibility in the care process.

Even in hospital environments, traditionally aimed at acute and corrective care, we see innovative experiences seeking to rescue patient vitality as part of treatment. The **Arts in Health at Duke** project integrates live music, artistic intervention, and sensory experiences into hospital care as part of the therapeutic plan. Reports indicate improved pain perception, reduced anxiety, and better clinical outcomes in critical patients.

In pediatric ICUs at Hospital Israelita Albert Einstein in São Paulo, a pioneering initiative adopted technologies like virtual reality to provide playful and relaxing experiences to children in intensive treatment. The idea was not just to entertain, but to reactivate desire, imagination, and autonomy fields in these children, thereby strengthening their coping processes. This fundamental objective of strengthening the organism to face a complex illness picture seems erased from thousands of hospitals in the country and world.

Potency also manifests when the system recognizes the cultural factor's importance. In a study conducted by University of Sydney researchers with Aboriginal populations, it became clear community health programs only worked when integrating elders' traditional knowledge and community rhythm into the clinical plan. Presence of local narratives, rituals, and practices increased adherence, activating feelings of belonging, value, and reciprocal care. The protocol ignoring culture also ignores potency.

Rethinking potency as a clinical resource is, ultimately, recognizing that what we amplify is sometimes more important than what we eliminate.

THEMATIC FOCUS: 6 DIMENSIONS OF HEALTH POTENCY

A model defining 6 forces sustaining health potency in anyone, even (or especially) in disease absence. This map is not metaphysical, nor "motivational." It is functional, clinical, and strategic, usable by professionals, platforms, technologies, or managers to understand, map, and promote health potency—before, during, or after any illness.

1. Relational Potency

❖ **What it represents:** Capacity to bond, trust, belong.
✷ **How it manifests:** Quality of bonds, presence of affective network, absence of chronic loneliness.
⊕ **How to cultivate clinically:** Care groups, active listening, social reintegration, bond prescription, social activities.

2. Rhythmic Potency

❖ **What it represents:** Capacity to maintain stable physiological and emotional rhythms.

✱ **How it manifests:** Restorative sleep, regulated appetite, healthy hormonal cycles, coherent cognitive flow.
⊕ **How to cultivate clinically:** Applied chronobiology, sleep hygiene, screen regulation, daily life ritualization.

3. Expressive Potency

❖ **What it represents:** Capacity to name emotions, create, mobilize meaning.
✱ **How it manifests:** Daily creativity, emotional freedom, affective vitality.
⊕ **How to cultivate clinically:** Integrative therapies, art as care, social/creative activities, self-reflection stimulus.

4. Adaptive Potency

❖ **What it represents:** Capacity to respond to change without collapsing.
✱ **How it manifests:** Emotional resilience, cognitive flexibility, reorientation in crises.
⊕ **How to cultivate clinically:** Support interventions in life transitions, narrative restructuring, body/nutrient strengthening.

5. Somatic Potency

❖ **What it represents:** Bodily energy available for action.
✱ **How it manifests:** Will to move, libido, physical disposition, high energy level.
⊕ **How to cultivate clinically:** Exercise/physical activity prescription, body reconnection, care for chronic pain/trauma.

6. Internal Coherence Potency

❖ **What it represents:** Feeling of alignment between personal trajectory, choices, and life direction.

✷ **How it manifests:** Clarity, sense of meaning, personal fulfillment.
⊕ **How to cultivate clinically:** Support for "self" reintegration: follow-up over time, expanded active listening, care accompanying patient over time (and between visits).

Traditional care asks: "What is wrong with you?". Potency-based care asks: "What is still strong, and how can we strengthen it further?"

~

These 6 dimensions were designed as a conceptual and didactic artifact for the book, anchored in disciplines:

- **Relational Potency:** ◬ Polyvagal Theory, Gabor Maté, attachment.
- **Rhythmic Potency:** ◬ Chronobiology, sleep, hormonal rhythmicity.
- **Expressive Potency:** ◬ Positive psychology, affective regulation, neuroaesthetics.
- **Adaptive Potency:** ◬ Emotional resilience, coping, neuroplasticity.
- **Somatic Potency:** ◬ Movement neurophysiology, vital tone, embodiment.
- **Internal Coherence Potency:** ◬ Antonovsky, Viktor Frankl, narrative medicine.

HEALTH AS FIELD OF CREATION, NOT MAINTENANCE

We arrive at a central point: potency is not an abstraction to be poeticized outside the office, but a legitimate, valuable clinical resource, often more decisive than isolated "technical" conduct. Ignoring it is wasting one of the most powerful tools we have to generate true health. And incorporating it does not mean abandoning science, but completing it with what makes it science—incorporating new findings, even if implying an effort to deeply reorganize practice.

And perhaps the most urgent step to make this possible is to demedicalize the clinical gaze, in the sense of freeing the professional from the diagnostic prison preventing them from seeing what is before them: a person, with stories, strengths, afflictions, dreams, and a living biography needing care. What would be possible if we recognized health as a field of active construction rather than just preservation?

This understanding considerably shifts the function of care from how it is practiced today. The health professional ceases to be the firefighter and becomes a construction partner, someone accompanying cycles, detours, trajectory leaps. This is much more complex than maintaining what already exists, but increased world complexity is here for everyone—for better or worse.

An elderly person who, at 82, decides to start painting classes and starts sleeping better, laughing more, talking to neighbors, and abandoning anxiolytics. A fibromyalgia patient who, after starting improv theater, reduces pain episodes, recovers emotional autonomy, and regains body confidence. An adolescent diagnosed with ADHD who, invited to co-create a school garden, experiences for the first time a sense of belonging, purpose, and affective stability. These cases are expressions of a health that does not fit in exams.

Creative potency is also revealed in moments of identity reorganization, when a person assumes new roles, revisits priorities, transforms relationships. This is shown by research on life transitions conducted by the University of Chicago, associating existential ruptures (like divorces, retirements, or career changes) with unexpected peaks of perceived health, when accompanied by emotional support and reconnection with personal meaning. Change, when sustained by context, can be therapeutic. It reorganizes us into new versions of ourselves. And this type of health flourishes when there is space. As philosopher Vinciane Despret wrote, "it is not knowledge that heals, it is listening allowing the other to become different from what they imagined themselves to be." Health, in this sense, is the process of becoming—not maintaining.

In pediatrics, this view is already more incorporated. Initiatives like **Boston Children's Hospital**, including artists, occupational therapists, and full-time caregivers as part of the clinical team, show healthy child development includes playing, exploring, testing limits, imagining futures. And it is in this creation that the body organizes, language expands, brain circuits refine.

The WHO itself, in its Health 2020 report, recognizes public policies must go beyond disease prevention and seek to promote health as a resource for daily life. This means investing in urban environments inviting movement, schools cultivating bonds, public spaces inspiring belonging. Creating health is not and never was the office's task; it is the task of everywhere life happens. And the office also needs to incorporate this fact into its practice in a structured way.

CHAPTER 13
THE HEALTH PROFESSIONALS IN THE CARE JOURNEY OF THE FUTURE

INVISIBLE IN DISCOURSE, INDISPENSABLE IN PRACTICE

Health discourses and imagery tend to concentrate around doctors, hospitals, and medicines. This trinity has shaped popular imagination, public policy, investments, and the very structure of health systems. But the everyday reality of care is infinitely broader, more plural, more interdependent. And in it, professionals such as nurses, nursing technicians, psychologists, physical therapists, occupational therapists, nutritionists, speech therapists, pharmacists, physical educators, community agents, caregivers, and social workers sustain, with little recognition, people's health.

These characters, despite being the absolute majority in the sector, continue to be invisible in strategic decisions, in spaces of power, in public representations, and even in dominant scientific literature. A simple search for articles with the word "nursing" or "enfermagem" in prestigious biomedical journals still reveals an abyss of visibility compared to the medical category. Knowledge production, when it exists, often circulates in niche journals with lower impact factors.

The organization of health work itself, especially in Brazil and other countries with a biomedical model, is structured around a hierarchy that still confuses authority with superiority. Instead of recognizing complementary competencies, the system frequently operates as a rigid pyramid, where medical knowledge occupies the top, followed by other professions in layers of subordination. This generates tensions among teams and compromises the collective intelligence of care.

Data from the Federal Council of Nursing show that Brazil has more than 2.7 million nursing professionals, including assistants, technicians, and graduated nurses, being the largest health workforce in the country. Despite the importance of this category, nursing still faces low remuneration, exhausting shifts, high psychosocial risks, and little space for clinical decision-making. During the COVID-19 pandemic, nurses were the ones who fell mentally ill the most, according to research by Fiocruz (2021), and also the ones who were most exposed and remained at the forefront of direct care.

The reality is not much different for other categories. Primary care psychologists work in contexts of high social complexity, deal with violence, family crises, chronic psychological suffering, and extreme vulnerabilities, frequently with precarious contracts, high turnover, and absence of clinical supervision. Hospital physical therapists, who are key players in the recovery of critically ill patients, are still treated by many managers as an additional cost. Occupational therapists, despite being fundamental in neurological rehabilitation, geriatrics, and mental health, face lack of knowledge even among health colleagues.

This devaluation has deep cultural roots. The figure of the doctor as the "holder of knowledge" was consolidated historically not only by their university education but by the way society constructed the symbolic authority of medicine. In a very different situation, nursing professionals were for decades associated with "care" functions, seen as less technical—a remnant of the patriarchal logic associating care with servitude. This stigma still persists in part of the population and in institutional environments. Just look at any public tender and compare the salaries for positions of doctor, nurse, psychologist, and so on. The difference is quite considerable.

But it is precisely this place of care that reveals the transformative strength of these professionals. While the biomedical model operates with a focus on disease, these professionals live with the patient in their entirety: they observe mood, perceive rhythm, detect subtle state variations, listen to anxieties that do not fit in the medical record. The nurse who notices a different look, the occupational therapist who perceives a regression gesture, the nutritionist who perceives an emotional relationship with food, all of them practice a refined clinic, but little recognized institutionally. Here, there is a latent opportunity, potentiated by the consolidation of emerging technologies, to systematically increase care multidisciplinarity, with increased strategic participation of these professionals throughout the entire patient journey.

Brazil still lacks a robust national policy formally integrating health professionals as strategy protagonists. Although the SUS (Unified Health System) recognizes multiprofessional work as ideal, in practice, many municipalities maintain rigid structures where only the doctor and the head nurse have a deliberative voice. Psychologists are called when there is a "problem," nutritionists are summoned to "correct diet," and occupational therapists are often not even included in teams.

The experience of countries valuing interdisciplinary models shows a different path. In Canada, primary care centers adopt the *Family Health Teams* model, in which doctors, nurses, nutritionists, psychologists, and pharmacists share clinical decisions in real time. Authority is diluted into competence, and the result is more integral care, less medicalized, and with lower public spending. What counts there is not the medical license stamp, but the capacity to listen, act, and collaborate.

It is fundamental to recognize that this invisibility has concrete consequences. Professionals with lower institutional recognition face more burnout, less autonomy, and higher turnover, which harms care continuity. According to the *The State of the World's Nursing 2020* report by the WHO, there is a direct correlation between professional valorization, team stability, and positive clinical outcomes. Heard and respected professionals care better because they also feel cared for.

In the context of mental health, the presence of diverse professionals is even more crucial. The Brazilian experience with CAPS (Psychosocial Care Centers) shows that it is precisely the presence of nursing technicians, occupational therapists, and psychologists in patients' daily lives that creates the relational space necessary for care.

Another emblematic example comes from experiences in indigenous health in Brazil, where indigenous health agents, traditional midwives, and professionals from the community itself play an essential role in cultural mediation of care. They are the ones making dialogue possible between technical knowledge and ancestral knowledge, and without them, the system simply does not function. But these figures remain underpaid, poorly trained institutionally, and rarely included in the teams' most strategic decisions.

Pharmacists, too, despite their highly specialized technical training, are underutilized. A study published in the *Revista Panamericana de Salud Pública* showed that the presence of the clinical pharmacist in primary care reduces medication-related adverse events and improves therapeutic adherence, especially among patients with chronic diseases. Yet, many managers treat them as simple "stock clerks" of supplies, ignoring their clinical potential.

Speech therapists and physical educators, in turn, are frequently perceived as "support services" rather than pillars of rehabilitation and prevention. This, despite robust evidence linking early intervention by these professionals to functional gains, reduced hospitalizations, and increased patient autonomy, especially in aging populations, with neurological diseases or developmental disorders. The invisibility of their clinical function is, first and foremost, a strategic waste.

Community health agents are another relevant case. Created to bring the SUS closer to peripheries and vulnerable communities, these professionals live at the intersection between the institutional and the everyday. They are the ones entering homes, listening to stories, identifying sufferings that were not verbalized. And despite this, they face fragile contracts, overload, violence risks, and often the disdain of professionals who see them as unqualified assistants. Brazil has tens of thousands of community agents active today. How many times are their voices heard in decisions?

Over time, this structure generated a double suffering: for patients, who do not feel heard, and for professionals, who cannot exercise their potency. Both fall ill. The consequence is a technically robust but symbolically impoverished system that simply does not solve the health crisis. And it is precisely for this reason that many of these professionals, even being passionate about their vocation, consider abandoning the area, seeking other professions, or accepting precarious positions.

HEALTH PROFESSIONALS WHO SUSTAIN PRESENCE

There is a listening that is learned in time, in subtle observation, in living with life's complexity. This listening happens at the bedside, in a patient's unexpected return, in a conversation interrupted for a tear, in the uncomfortable silence between news and a reaction. It is this listening that many health professionals, especially those accompanying the patient with more constancy and less technical apparatus, develop.

Nurses, nursing technicians, occupational therapists, psychologists, physical therapists, community agents, and so many other professionals are where care happens when the doctor has already left the room. They perceive what was not said, notice variations exams do not show, recognize emotional, family, relational patterns. Professor and psychotherapist Carl Rogers already stated that genuine, empathetic, present listening is therapeutic in itself. In his person-centered approach, he demonstrated that the simple fact of someone feeling heard, in a non-judgmental way and with true presence, mobilizes internal processes of reorganization, self-regulation, and even healing. Rogers said listening is the soil where transformation is born. And in health, this becomes visible in simple and clinically potent gestures.

A nurse noticing the patient no longer touches food, although saying they are fine; a health agent noting the elderly lady stopped watering her plants, although denying sadness; a physical therapist hearing the exaggerated effort in how someone says "it's all good"—it is in these details that health reveals itself in its most sensitive layer. And, if welcomed with presence, these signs can be more diagnostic than any imaging exam.

French psychologist Boris Cyrulnik, studying resilience paths, showed that the first protective factor in people who went through great traumas was the presence of someone who listened to them welcomingly. Listening saves, reorganizes, treats. Anyone who has been in a hospital, public or private, has seen the time the doctor usually spends in contact with the patient in the room, and knows it may not exceed 2 minutes a day, not as an exception, but as a completely institutionalized practice that, apparently, does not violate medical ethics. Let's be pragmatic: there is much more listening practice being practiced by nurses than doctors, on average. And here lies a treasure clinical practice will still learn to leverage much more—and acceleratedly with technologies enabling a more continuous and broad view of the patient.

This is why many of these professionals frequently report becoming "confidants," "escape valves," "safe harbors" for their patients. But this function is often seen as a waste of time, as "too much talk," as something escaping clinical focus, and this devaluation falls on the professional themselves. A nursing technician spending nights monitoring a patient's pain but not included in case discussion, or a psychologist identifying a recurrent emotional pattern in a chronic patient but having no space to present their reading to the team.

In a study conducted by the Federal University of Santa Catarina with primary care professionals, nursing technicians reported feeling emotionally exhausted by accumulating the listening function for patients and other team members, without having a space to care for themselves. Listening is a gift, but it also needs listening back. Otherwise, the professional implodes.

Most moving is that, even without formal recognition, many of these professionals know the value of listening. And continue exercising this care with dignity, creativity, and presence. Because they know the soul of care is there. A physical therapist reported, at a congress, spending three weeks accompanying a quadriplegic patient without achieving any motor progress. But, at the end, he told her: "You were the only person who made me feel alive in this hospital." Sometimes, that is everything.

The systems working best are those that knew how to organize care around presence. Qualified listening precedes prescription. It guides, aligns, sensitizes. And when incorporated with awareness, the system itself becomes more sensible and efficient.

THE SILENCED HEALTH PROFESSIONAL

Despite being decisive in care continuity and being among the first to capture subtle changes in a patient's state, professionals like nurses, physical therapists, occupational therapists, psychologists, nutritionists, pharmacists, and community health agents continue facing deep structural obstacles limiting their clinical potency. These obstacles are expressions of a historically doctor-centric system, which shaped forms of invisibility continuing to operate even when discourse favors integrality. The result is an impoverishing paradox (yes, we will confront many paradoxes throughout the work): the professionals closest to the patient's daily life are also those whose perceptions and knowledges are most blocked or disregarded by clinical decision structures.

This blockage happens in multiple layers, and a study, "Multiprofessional Teamwork in Primary Care: Barriers and Facilitators," interviewing more than 300 primary care professionals in four countries, identified the constant presence of implicit hierarchies in clinical decisions, even in contexts self-declaring interdisciplinary. According to data, nurses reported having their observations about the patient frequently discarded by doctors, even when these observations involved relevant clinical alerts. This exclusion of technical listening frustrates the professional and compromises the clinical outcome. As a nurse participating in the study stated: "You can be saying pain is worsening, breathing pattern changed, but if it doesn't come with the right signature, no one listens."

This type of erasure was also identified by Brazilian researchers in the ObservaRH project (Fiocruz, 2021), where physical therapists and occupational therapists in the public network reported recurrent experience of being called to "do motor rehabilitation" or "playful activities," even when identifying, in daily life, cognitive alterations, early signs of depression, or broader functional impairment. The report shows about 60% of these professionals stated not being invited to team meetings or therapeutic plan construction, despite accompanying patients more frequently than other team members.

This absence of space is directly linked to legal and institutional structures treating clinical practice as an exclusive prerogative of medicine. The discussion about the "medical act," widely debated in Brazil after approval of Law 12.842/2013, clearly exposed the conflict between multiprofessional clinical practices and a corporate logic seeking to preserve medical authority as the only legitimate reference. The Medical Act Law defined which acts are exclusive to doctors, such as disease diagnosis and treatment prescription. Some parts of the law were vetoed by the Presidency, especially the one making nosological diagnosis (disease identification) an exclusive act of doctors. This veto was made to avoid harm to public health programs where other professionals, like nurses, already act based on established protocols. The veto does not give authorization to other health professionals to diagnose diseases autonomously, only preserves what was already provided for in respective professions' laws.

But even though legislation suffered important vetoes, it produced a silent side effect: institutional fear. Professionals began reporting legal insecurity to exercise activities involving assessment, non-pharmacological conduct prescription, or participation in therapeutic decisions. COFFITO (Federal Council of Physical Therapy and Occupational Therapy) expresses concerns about professional restriction. This fear comes from how the law is interpreted and operationalized within institutions. It is common to find managers restricting nutritionists' attributions to providing standardized diets, even when these professionals have training and could act on therapeutic adherence of chronic patients.

In many services, case discussion moments center on the medical agenda, with little or no space for other professionals to bring their clinical perceptions. Even when team meetings are held, as in the Family Health Teams model, various studies point out that therapeutic plan construction remains dominated by a verticalized logic. According to ENSP/Fiocruz research (2022), conducted with 400 professionals in Basic Health Units of four Brazilian capitals, 65% of non-medical professionals reported their suggestions on patient clinical management were "frequently ignored or disregarded." The most reported feeling was "being on the team, but not part of the decision."

In many medical records, especially digitized ones, fields dedicated to non-medical professionals are restricted to operational records or administrative observations, preventing their clinical interpretations from becoming part of therapeutic reasoning. A physical therapist cannot record that the patient "expressed emotional resistance to movement," an occupational therapist finds no space to report "insecurity regarding return home," and a community health agent has nowhere to insert the report that "the patient cried and trembled when talking about her husband, but said it was just tiredness." What has no field has no value.

In a report by nurse Mariana Floriano, published in the book

"Clínica Comum" (2021), she describes how, after months being unauthorized by a manager when proposing changes in a public hospital's palliative care routine, she started recording the minimum in the chart. This type of giving up is corrosive and also felt by patients. In qualitative research conducted by UFMG (2020) with chronic patients treated by multiprofessional teams, various interviewees said they "trusted more who was always there." But when asked if this professional decided the treatment, everyone said no.

Despite this, blocking these professionals' potency hasn't prevented it from manifesting. In many services, these are the professionals creating silent strategies to sustain the bond: calling to see how the patient is, adjusting conduct to the person's way of life, making informal articulations with support networks. These practices do not appear in productivity reports, but they prevent the collapse of many bonds. And even if the system doesn't recognize them, the patient does—and is grateful.

Faced with all this, it is not enough for institutional discourse to speak of multidisciplinarity. It is necessary to reconstruct structures operating this discourse: listening, medical records, governance, legality, remuneration, flow, language. It is not little, just as the cases of people in suffering missing out on better health due to lack of support for decisive professionals in this journey are not few.

THEMATIC FOCUS: ONE BODY, VARIOUS LENSES - WHAT EACH PROFESSIONAL REALLY SEES WHEN ENTERING THE ROOM

The same patient. The same symptom. But 8 completely different interpretations—all correct.

This chart simulates the same patient entering a consultation room, but being seen by different professionals, revealing how each training, approach, and clinical framework sees fragments of the same human being complementarily and not necessarily convergently.

Patient: Woman, 39, works in corporate environment, presents diffuse body pain, persistent tiredness, irregular sleep, irritability, altered menstrual cycle, lab tests within normal limits.

General Practitioner

👁🗨 **What they see first:** Tiredness and pain without lab alteration.
💬 **How they interpret:** "Functional picture. Could be stress or something somatoform."
⚕ **Typical conduct (isolated):** Prescribes mild symptomatics, orders new blood count.
🔎 **Missing without other lenses:** Ignores emotional cycle, habits, gut, bond.

Endocrinologist

👁🗨 **What they see first:** Hormonal irregularity and fatigue.
💬 **How they interpret:** "May be mild thyroid dysfunction, even with normal TSH."
⚕ **Typical conduct (isolated):** Evaluates T3/T4, proposes eventual hormone replacement.
🔎 **Missing without other lenses:** Does not treat sleep, bond, or emotion—focuses on hormonal axis.

Clinical Psychologist

👁🗨 **What they see first:** Irritability, tension, dissatisfaction.
💬 **How they interpret:** "Narrative of unmetabolized emotional overload."
⚕ **Typical conduct (isolated):** Active listening, support, naming conflict.
🔎 **Missing without other lenses:** Does not act on dietary patterns, sleep, or physical.

Functional Nutritionist

👁️🗨️ **What they see first:** Binge peak, post-meal tiredness, oscillating gut.
💬 **How they interpret:** "Mild inflammatory picture due to diet and dysbiosis."
⚕️ **Typical conduct (isolated):** Dietary adjustment, gut flora care.
🔎 **Missing without other lenses:** Does not access trauma, bond, or emotional perception.

Physical Educator

👁️🗨️ **What they see first:** Body rigidity and chronic tiredness.
💬 **How they interpret:** "Disuse and inactivity perpetuate muscle fatigue."
⚕️ **Typical conduct (isolated):** Introduces progressive movement plan.
🔎 **Missing without other lenses:** Can aggravate if ignoring emotional exhaustion or chronic pain.

Physical Therapist

👁️🗨️ **What they see first:** Compensatory postural patterns, myofascial blocks.
💬 **How they interpret:** "Picture of accumulated tension, without adequate release."
⚕️ **Typical conduct (isolated):** Manual therapy, breathing, body awareness.
🔎 **Missing without other lenses:** Does not access emotional narrative or work environment role.

Occupational Therapist

👁️🗨️ **What they see first:** Drop in daily functionality and time management.

💬 **How they interpret:** "Misalignment between routine and functional capacity."
⚕ **Typical conduct (isolated):** Rhythm redesign, autonomy rescue.
🔎 **Missing without other lenses:** Isolatedly, may not interfere in internal illness factors.

Nurse (with expanded listening)

👁 🗨 **What they see first:** Life rhythm, self-care habits, adherence to conduct.
💬 **How they interpret:** "Patient who cares for everyone, but not herself."
⚕ **Typical conduct (isolated):** Counseling, health education, trust bond.
🔎 **Missing without other lenses:** Lacks diagnostic decision power, but sustains trust.

> EVERYONE IS RIGHT—WITHIN THEIR LENS. THE PROBLEM IS WHEN THE LENS BECOMES A BORDER. THE CARE JOURNEY BEGINS WHEN THESE LENSES OVERLAP, LISTEN, CHALLENGE, AND INTERTWINE. BECAUSE NO PATIENT IS JUST A PAIN, A SYMPTOM, AN EXAM. THEY ARE A SET OF VECTORS ONLY UNDERSTANDABLE BY A SET OF GAZES.

MULTIDISCIPLINARY PROTAGONISM IN FUTURE HEALTHCARE

When looking closely at moments when professionals usually sidelined in clinical hierarchies gain space to work more freely, it becomes clear care style changes. It is a change in system intelligence itself, and effects are measurable.

At Hospital Sírio-Libanês, a clinical reorganization experience started from the rehabilitation sector. Instead of keeping physical therapists and occupational therapists as medical plan execution arms, the hospital repositioned them as coordinators of post-ICU rehabilitation trajectories. Based on international evidence on post-intensive care syndrome, they began leading conduct centered on patient functionality and reintegration into daily life. The *Revista Brasileira de Terapias Cognitivas* documented significant quality of life improvement in patients in 3 months, with reduced average length of stay and autonomy gains.

Professionals like occupational therapists, when leading meaning reconstruction projects in mental health centers, manage to access layers not even the most attentive psychiatrist could address alone.

The Institute of Physical Medicine and Rehabilitation at Hospital das Clínicas built a post-COVID rehabilitation model based on integrated action of physical therapists, speech therapists, psychologists, and occupational therapists. These professionals, instead of waiting for medical referral, organized motor, cognitive, and emotional rehabilitation axes among themselves based on functional history and each patient's rhythm.

And professionals report increased work meaning, reduced emotional exhaustion, and improved inter-team cooperation. In a survey by the Regional Psychology Council of São Paulo (Brazil), interviewees working in teams with shared clinical decisions reported greater satisfaction with professional practice and feeling of recognition. When the clinic is truly shared, every listening becomes reorganization possibility. This is health beginning to sketch itself as a new possible horizon.

THE FUTURE IS TRANSDISCIPLINARY: COLLECTIVE INTELLIGENCE IN HEALTH

The emergence of a new care model, more collaborative, transversal, and sensitive to life facts is a concrete possibility, based both on new available technologies and clinical practices already happening out there. But for this to be the rule, not exception, logic of clinical centralization must shift, substituting old decision monopoly with collective intelligence already pulsing, even at margins, in so many multidisciplinary teams. And this shift needs to be structured, sustained, legitimized, operationalized.

Technologies like Internet of Things (IoT), wearable sensors, integrated records, clinical data dashboards, and connected health apps made possible something previously unimaginable: continuous monitoring of patient health state by multiple professionals, from multiple areas, with shared data access and possibility of immediate coordinated action. These tools' potential depends less on technical sophistication and more on how they are used: to concentrate (and limit), or distribute care power.

In a collaboration-centered system, as health will be in a few years (whether we like it or not), these data become legitimate input for different professionals to exercise clinical autonomy. A physical therapist can propose adaptations in home rehabilitation plan based on sleep and activity patterns collected by mobile devices. A nutritionist can evaluate metabolic effects of meal plan more precisely based on connected daily glucose data. A psychologist can monitor mood patterns and build early interventions to prevent relapses.

Digitization can be bridge between knowledges. But only if there is clear political decision first: that healthcare is plural by nature and must be built by those actually sustaining daily care. Case coordination can change according to journey moment, respecting complexity and quantity of factors involved: pharmacists leading multiple medication interventions; physical therapists assuming chronic pain patients; social workers coordinating support strategies in vulnerability contexts.

ConecteSUS represents one of largest health interoperability efforts ever made. In municipalities where system is well operated, like Aracaju and Vitória da Conquista, community agents can register sensitive situations, and this information reaches clinical team without distortion. This allows decisions based on evidence going beyond office, and health agent ceases to be info passer to become territory analyst.

Integration between clinical data and qualified listening of these professionals opens space for more responsive clinic. Imagine team where nursing technician notices, from home visit, elderly patient has less social interaction. This information, combined with drop in physical activity levels captured by sensors, can lead physical therapist and occupational therapist to propose expanded rehabilitation plan before clinical decompensation or avoidable hospitalization occurs. This already happening in diverse health units in São Paulo interior.

Possibilities opened by AI-based predictive systems also gain clinical potency if used by different human listeners. Algorithm can indicate increased heart failure hospitalization risk, but who interprets this risk with density, considering patient affective adherence, family history, housing conditions, and moment's emotional complexity, are frontline professionals.

Interdisciplinarity becomes more operational when technology favors flow. Instead of isolated records, professionals start writing in common language, building joint reasoning, revising conduct transparently. Occupational therapist doesn't write for herself, but for team. Pharmacist doesn't point problem, but proposes joint solution. Care ceases to be sum of reports and becomes collective construction.

Use of integrated electronic records, like Tasy, facilitates exchange. System allows different health professionals access to real-time patient info, share notes, define joint care plans, monitor clinical evolution coordinately. Patients themselves also become care agents. Chronic disease patients using apps to log symptoms, mood variations, sleep patterns, or eating habits often discover correlations with professionals they'd never perceive alone.

Digital transformation alone doesn't democratize health. Must be accompanied by institutional transformation recognizing clinical value of those always close to patient. Requires changing team meetings, decision flows, remuneration, continuing education, and above all changing imaginary of who can be clinician. And not enough to call everyone to table—must listen and legitimize. Difference now is collaboration can rely on systems documenting, connecting, articulating, preventing precious observations from getting lost.

Pandemic accelerated process. Rehabilitation professionals previously acting locally started monitoring patients via telecare, creating hybrid care protocols mixing in-person observation, remote logging, collective decision making. In many networks, enabled care continuity. Managers understanding this are redesigning protocols. In Belo Horizonte, Municipal Health Secretariat created digital interdisciplinary flows where each professional, logging data, automatically triggers others. Final decision belongs to consensus of those knowing different patient layers. And this directly impacting readmission rates, falling in pilot units.

Same movement happening in private networks. Hospitals like Albert Einstein and HCor investing in clinical platforms integrating physiotherapy, nutrition, clinical pharmacy, psychology, medicine decisions. These teams' performance—and patients'—improved. Because professionals repositioned as central agents of care strategy.

Most updated universities including interprofessional practice disciplines with simulations based on integrated records and shared real cases. Future of healthcare being trained not as vertical, but horizontal. And this will reflect, in few years, in how health systems operate. Future clinic will necessarily be presence clinic articulated by data, where algorithm helps better direct listening and sensor doesn't eliminate conversation but prepares it. Where professionals from different areas don't compete for authority but lean on each other to sustain care in its complexity. And when knowing observations considered, write better, listen more, expose themselves with more courage. Record quality improves and clinical analysis gains depth.

Doesn't mean conflict absence. Real teams have tensions, limits, disputes. But shared data, care plan, trust built between professionals allow tensions to be productive, not paralyzing. What was space dispute can become listening tuning. This is institutional maturity and system as whole wins, because with co-responsibility errors fall, adherence rises, costs decrease, results sustain. International literature categorical here: well-operated interprofessional clinic more efficient than segmented clinic. And now, with digital resources, also more possible.

Protagonism of non-medical health professionals is not concession: it is condition for clinic to sustain itself. That's what data shows, cases reveal, patients feel. And that's what most attentive managers already incorporating in policies and decisions.

In some networks, already consolidated reality. In others, still struggle. At stake is system efficiency and dignity of professionals sustaining health every day. Technology can, finally, return to these professionals what was always theirs: place at clinic center.

And work you are reading is detailed construction about this: how to make care practice of distributed, sensitive intelligence, where each professional is more than executor and each patient more than receiver. This is new clinic starting to emerge: technological, yes. But deeply human. And, precisely for this, more potent than any isolated algorithm or underused new technology could ever be.

CHAPTER 14
THE CHALLENGE OF SUSTAINING HEALTH

THE CONCEPT OF REGENERATION: NOT JUST TREATING, BUT SUSTAINING HEALTH

When we speak of regenerative health, we are referring to a clinical and systemic logic based on the finding that life is movement, and that care implies sustaining conditions for the organism to reorganize its own balances, dynamics, and adaptations; it is creating fertile ground for vitality to happen.

This is already present in various scientific fronts and clinical practices, in an increasingly articulated way. In cellular biology, studies demonstrate that the human body repairs and reconfigures its functions based on continuous interaction with internal and external stimuli. In the field of regenerative medicine, therapies with stem cells, tissue bioprinting, and molecular engineering already demonstrate that regeneration is a scientific frontier.

But the concept goes beyond the molecular level and extends to the systemic level of care: regenerating means building support networks that favor the plasticity of the organism and subjectivity in the face of adversities. It means considering that the subject falls ill in cycles, in contexts, in non-linear dynamics, and that the clinical proposal cannot be limited to erasing symptoms; it needs to offer tools, environments, and relationships that sustain the continuous reorganization process, including to be more economically viable in the long term.

Lifestyle medicine is one of the areas closest to this logic. Various studies have long demonstrated that interventions in sleep, diet, physical activity, stress management, and interpersonal relationships prevent diseases and also reverse chronic conditions previously considered irreversible.

And this terrain is, largely, relational. Psychology, especially in integrative and systemic approaches, already recognizes that a subject's emotional reorganization depends less on eliminating traumas and more on building new networks of sustenance, belonging, and meaning. Psychotherapy models like Internal Family Systems, Acceptance and Commitment Therapy, and compassion-based mindfulness practices act to expand the subject's internal regeneration capacity in the face of pain.

Functional medicine also rests on this idea. By seeking to identify imbalances behind clinical manifestations, it proposes therapeutic plans prioritizing the restoration of the intestinal axis, mitochondrial metabolism, and immunomodulation. But perhaps where the idea of regeneration becomes most powerful is in the articulation between the clinical dimension and the environmental dimension (in the broad sense of the word).

From a technological point of view, regeneration also becomes more possible with advances in real-time data analysis, personalized genomics, integration between environmental signals and physiological variables, continuous sensorization, predictive algorithms applied to health, AI agents, and even gamification. A system capturing micro-variations in heart rate, respiratory patterns, glucose levels, and peripheral temperature can anticipate decompensations and allow early interventions, guided by that organism's specific patterns. The so-called 5P Medicine —personalized, predictive, preventive, participatory, and precision— also aligns with this movement. Instead of waiting for the disease to set in, it seeks to identify vulnerabilities, interpret patterns, and act on multiple levels.

Sustaining, moreover, is a verb needing revaluation in the clinic. Sustaining is being present even when there is no quick fix, accompanying the patient in their time, offering qualified presence, active listening, adaptation. Regeneration demands time to observe, adapt, trust, try again, learn to do differently. From an organizational standpoint, it demands flows favoring the patient's return to care whenever necessary, without this being interpreted as failure. On the contrary: returning is an opportunity to express trust, the sense of continuity.

WE ARE LIVING A HISTORICAL MOMENT

We have reached a point in history where the possibility of transforming healthcare into something deep, continuous, and regenerative is a reality. We live a kind of sophisticated mismatch: a system operating with extremely advanced technologies in some sectors and with others quite outdated and worse than those of other markets.

We are not claiming the health sector is technologically backward—that would be imprecise. What happens is a lag between existing technical potential and how this potential is incorporated into care practices, flows, and social commitments. Technology is present. Scientific knowledge is there to guide it. And it is not always expensive. What is missing is clinical rooting, institutional maturity, and ethical clarity on how these tools should be used to generate health and not just procedural efficiency or a better late correction.

Why, even with all these resources, do we continue failing in the most fundamental indicators of collective health? Why do chronicity, avoidable suffering, hospital turnover, judicialization, patient feelings of abandonment, and professional burnout increase? Do we not, each of us, have the responsibility not only to understand this but to position ourselves as patients and professionals who see better paths exist, and demand things that today are already the minimum, not a differential?

Most health institutions, public or private, clinical or hospital, regulatory or operational, are still trapped in a logic of productivity, fragmentation, and legal defense, and this is productive for (almost) no one. Data is collected to justify actions, not to build bonds or intelligence. Platforms are designed for auditing, not listening. Hello? Good morning! Shall we talk about obvious things that can no longer be treated as normal?

Public policies, remuneration models, quality indicators, and clinical decision flows still operate under a logic of events, not trajectory. We are often sophisticating what should have already been overcome (considering technical capacity, scientific knowledge, and patient well-being), and calling it transformation.

At the same time, we see emerging, at this system's limits, a new type of social intelligence. Health professionals seeking autonomy to create more sensitive care plans and current disciplines integrating patient lifestyle and narrative as fundamental input. Patients demanding more participation and transparency. Families organizing into support networks. Digital platforms promoting self-care, education, remote monitoring, and collective knowledge construction. New professionals with diversified knowledge.

Integral care is spoken of, but isolated productivity is funded. Active listening is spoken of, but the consultation is timed in a few minutes. Cutting-edge technology is spoken of, but where algorithms are most used is in anti-fraud mechanisms to deny procedures. This abyss between discourse and practice will not be solved with more technology but with new demands, curricular revision and quality control of university courses, and the action of people like you who want and can do and speak about better paths—and things we cannot pretend are pro-health.

The State also needs to position itself as a financier and strategic articulator of effective intersectoral and transdisciplinary policies, holistically considering the complex web of social determinants of health. It is no longer useful to launch fragmented health programs if urbanization logic continues favoring exclusionary and unsustainable models not thought for people, if the food production chain adopts ultra-processed standards known to be harmful to health without adequate package warnings, or if health professionals' working conditions maintain precarious and exhausting dynamics.

Health will only be regenerative when at the center of public policy, guiding decisions in areas like transport, housing, education, and environment. The example of cities adopting the "Health in All Policies" concept, like Helsinki and Toronto, demonstrates this approach is not utopian.

In Brazil, initiatives in cities like Curitiba, with its integrated urban planning and focus on green areas, show positive results in population quality of life. Integrating health into public policies is viable and beneficial in different socioeconomic contexts. Thus, it is imperative that health ceases to be treated as a separate sector, limited to disease management, and becomes a central structuring axis of public policies.

Universities and training centers, likewise, need to exit the rhetoric of "innovation" and assume their responsibility in training professionals who operate the clinic of the future. This means preparing to deal with complexity, uncertainty, listening, conversational AI, not just procedures (which will increasingly be replaceable by autonomous technologies and AI...). And it means building bridges between disciplines, between knowledges. Knowledge needs to stop being vertical to become transversal. And, on this path, it needs to recruit other knowledges and other professionals: designers, software developers, psychologists, product managers, data scientists, biomedical scientists, and so on.

And if there is, at this moment, a misguided narrative still reigning in many decision-making circles, it is that shifting to a smarter, continuous, and humane care model would be too expensive, slow, or uncertain. The truth, sustained by abundant evidence, is exactly the opposite: maintaining the current system is what costs dearly. Insisting on fragmentation, repetition of unnecessary exams, avoidable readmissions, lack of coordination, discontinuity of care plans generates a cycle of immense waste, judicialization, and structural inefficiency compromising the system's sustainability as a whole.

But what perhaps has not yet become sufficiently clear is that this new model also represents a huge market opportunity for all involved. Health technology companies managing to align their solutions with this regenerative logic will have more adherence to a hyperconnected market, more impact, more loyalty. Hospitals migrating from volume-centered to value-centered models will be more sustainable. Health plans understanding that prevention and bonding are sources of savings will have competitive advantage. Professionals positioning themselves as trajectory managers, not mere procedure executors, will have protagonism and preference.

Society is changing faster than systems. People already expect more transparency, continuity, autonomy, listening. They already live connected, already monitor their own bodies, already seek qualified information, already share experiences. There is a mismatch between health culture and society culture. And this mismatch is, simultaneously, a problem and an opportunity. Whoever knows how to occupy this vacuum with intelligence, integrity, and competence will lead the transformation, and grow with it.

This also applies to the public system. Adopting more integrated, territorial, sensitive, and digitally articulated models can radically improve public policy effectiveness, optimize resources, and increase population trust in the SUS. Successful experiences in cities like Recife, Vitória da Conquista, and Aracaju show it is possible to articulate surveillance, primary care, mental health, and emergency data with intelligent protocols and qualified listening. Gains are clinical, but also political: a system that listens is a system that rebuilds legitimacy.

The market is understanding that true disruption lies in redesigning the care path based on bonding, vectors, data, and regeneration. This demands another type of intelligence overflowing medicine, just as it overflows technology, psychology, design, neuroscience.

There is also a decisive role for funders: banks, investment funds, multilateral organizations, fiscal incentives. Capital needs to understand that investing in regenerative health is investing in social stability, economic productivity, population resilience. The return is financial too. A country with fewer chronic patients, less judicialization, less waste is a country with more fiscal margin, more workforce, more well-being.

Therefore, what this "book-chapter" proposes is a lens shift revealing that health is a construction. And that this construction needs, more than ever, explicit, generous, intelligent agreements committed to life regeneration.

What we began to do here, with references, cases, and ponderations, is place a magnifying glass to recognize these signals and propose they stop being exceptions.

Because we have never had so many resources, so much science, so much technology, and so much urgency to reorganize care, and we are at the beginning of the journey for a great turnaround in medicine.

ABOUT THE AUTHOR

João Guilherme Franco holds a degree in Communications and Advertising from the University of São Paulo (USP), an MBA in Internet of Things from Poli-USP, and a postgraduate credential in Strategic Marketing from Insper. A Marketing, Product Management, and Innovation executive with more than 22 years of experience, he has built a career developing services and strategies in markets that sit at the intersection of technology, behavior, design, language, and value creation.

His path is marked by an essentially transdisciplinary approach—born of a passion for connecting distinct, complementary perspectives and bodies of knowledge to "watch the magic happen." He has worked in insurance, technology companies, startups, and major enterprises such as BTG, Vivo, Michelin, and ClearSale. Today, he channels that experience toward his true passion: sparking deep change in how we see, design, and practice healthcare—exploring how new opportunities are, gradually (and sometimes not so gradually), reshaping one of the world's most complex and strategic domains: health.

Throughout his career, he has stood at the center of complex challenges that required not only creating value and differentiation but also ensuring demand and profitability for innovative services and solutions. Over the years, he has organized ideas and notes on the deep dysfunctions he studied and observed: payment models decoupled from patient outcomes; practices that ignore structural causes; and the fragmentation of care that leaves patients isolated amid tests, protocols, and disconnected data—a whole apparatus of procedures that does little to change the health landscape.

That discomfort grows sharper against the contrast between what is possible and what is systematically neglected by the insularity of clinical knowledge. We are at an inflection point: on one side, the traditional mechanistic model that insists on denying the complexity of interactions among body, emotions, environment, habits, and lifestyle; on the other, demonstrably more effective initiatives—capable of overcoming critical limits of conventional practice and extracting better value from professionals, technologies, and resources.

With intellectual independence, clarity, and no institutional ties that might narrow his view, João Guilherme Franco is committed to naming the "elephants in the room" that daily practice prefers to ignore—and that many training programs never even address. His aim is to provoke the fundamental conversations healthcare needs for its future—without romanticism or ornament—and, above all, to get to the core of the opportunities by pointing to concrete solutions that can be implemented now.

REFERENCES

CHAPTER 1

ANTONOVSKY, A. *Health, Stress, and Coping*. San Francisco: Jossey-Bass, 1979.

BARRATT, A. Overdiagnosis in mammography screening: a 45 year journey from shadowy idea to acknowledged reality. *BMJ*, v. 350, Mar. 2015. DOI: 10.1136/bmj.h867.

CANGUILHEM, G. *The Normal and the Pathological*. 5th ed. rev. exp. Rio de Janeiro: Forense Universitária, 2002.

CSIKSZENTMIHALYI, M. *Flow: The Psychology of Optimal Experience*. New York: Harper & Row, 1990.

DAMASIO, A. *Descartes' Error: Emotion, Reason, and the Human Brain*. Translated by Dora Vicente and Georgina Segurado. São Paulo: Companhia das Letras, 1996.

DESCARTES, R. *Meditations on First Philosophy*. São Paulo: WMF Martins Fontes, 2021.

ENGEL, G. L. The Need for a New Medical Model: A Challenge for Biomedicine. *Science*, v. 196, n. 4286, p. 129–136, 8 Apr. 1977. DOI: 10.1126/science.847460.

GRUNDY, Scott M., et al. Guideline on the Management of Blood Cholesterol: A Report of the American College of Cardiology/American Heart Association Task Force on Clinical Practice Guidelines. *Journal of the American College of Cardiology*, v. 73, n. 24, p. e285-e350, Jun. 2019. DOI: 10.1016/j.jacc.2018.11.003.

HORVATH, S. DNA methylation age of human tissues and cell types. *Genome Biology*, v. 14, n. 10, p. R115, 2013. DOI: 10.1186/gb-2013-14-10-r115.

INSTITUTE OF SUPPLEMENTARY HEALTH STUDIES (IESS). *Fraud and Waste in Supplementary Health*. Study conducted by EY. IESS, 2023. Available at: https://www.iess.org.br/biblioteca/tds-e-estudos/estudos-especiais-externos/fraudes-e-desperdicios-em-saude-suplementar

WU J, Gao X, Yang Z, Yang Y, Galea G, Wang L et al. Non-pharmacological interventions for prevention and treatment of non-communicable diseases with experiences from China. *BMJ*, 2024; 387:e076764. DOI:10.1136/bmj-2023-076764

MATURANA, H. R.; VARELA, F. J. *The Tree of Knowledge: The Biological Roots of Human Understanding*. São Paulo: Palas Athena, 2001.

MCEWEN, B. S. Physiology and Neurobiology of Stress and Adaptation: Central Role of the Brain. *Physiological Reviews*, v. 87, n. 3, p. 873–904, Jul. 2007. DOI: 10.1152/physrev.00041.2006.

MOSCATELLO, E. et al. Delayed diagnosis adversely affects outcome in systemic lupus erythematosus: Cross sectional analysis of the LuLa cohort. *PLoS One*, v. 16, n. 1, p. e0244783, 2021.

WORLD HEALTH ORGANIZATION (WHO). *Constitution of the World Health Organization*. New York: World Health Organization, 1946.

SALLNOW, L. et al. Report of the Lancet Commission on the Value of Death: bringing death back into life. *The Lancet*, v. 399, n. 10327, p. 837-884, 2022.
SELIGMAN, M. E. P. *Authentic Happiness: Using the New Positive Psychology to Realize Your Potential for Lasting Fulfillment*. New York: Free Press, 2002.
SHRANK, W. H.; ROGSTAD, T. L.; PAREKH, N. Waste in the US Health Care System: Estimated Costs and Potential for Savings. *JAMA*, v. 322, n. 15, p. 1501–1509, 2019. DOI: 10.1001/jama.2019.13978.
SUKHODOLSKY, D. G. et al. Traditional and atypical presentations of anxiety in youth with autism spectrum disorder. *Journal of Autism and Developmental Disorders*, v. 47, n. 6, p. 1773-1784, 2017.
VARELA, F. J.; THOMPSON, E.; ROSCH, E. *The Embodied Mind: Cognitive Science and Human Experience*. Cambridge, MA: MIT Press, 1991.
ZEEVI, D. et al. Personalized Nutrition by Prediction of Glycemic Responses. *Cell*, v. 163, n. 5, p. 1079–1094, 19 Nov. 2015. DOI: 10.1016/j.cell.2015.11.001.

CHAPTER 2

BLACKBURN, Elizabeth; EPEL, Elissa. *The Telomere Effect: A Revolutionary Approach to Living Younger, Healthier, Longer*. New York: Grand Central Publishing, 2017.
BROWNLEE, Shannon. *Overtreated: Why Too Much Medicine Is Making Us Sicker and Poorer*. New York: Bloomsbury Publishing, 2007.
CANGUILHEM, Georges. *The Normal and the Pathological*. 3rd ed. Rio de Janeiro: Forense Universitária, 1990.
CONRAD, Peter. *The Medicalization of Society: On the Transformation of Human Conditions into Treatable Disorders*. Baltimore: Johns Hopkins University Press, 2007.
COOTER, Roger; HARRISON, Mark; STURDY, Steve (ed.). *Medicine and modern warfare*. Amsterdam: Rodopi, 1999. (Clio medica, v. 55).
DAMASIO, Antonio R. *Descartes' Error: Emotion, Reason, and the Human Brain*. New York: GP Putnam, 1994.
FOUCAULT, Michel. *The Birth of the Clinic*. 7th ed. Rio de Janeiro: Forense Universitária, 2011. Translated by Roberto Machado.
FOX, Renée C. *Experiment Perilous: Physicians and Patients Facing the Unknown*. Rev. ed. New Brunswick: Transaction Publishers, 1998.
FRANCES, Allen. *Saving Normal: An Insider's Revolt Against Out-of-Control Psychiatric Diagnosis, DSM-5, Big Pharma, and the Medicalization of Ordinary Life*. 1st ed. New York: William Morrow, 2013.
GAWANDE, Atul. *Being Mortal: Medicine and What Matters in the End*. Rio de Janeiro: Objetiva, 2015. Translated by Renata Telles.
GØTZSCHE, Peter C. *Deadly Medicines and Organised Crime: How Big Pharma Has Corrupted Healthcare*. London: Radcliffe Publishing, 2013.
GREENHALGH, Trisha et al. Evidence based medicine: a movement in crisis? *BMJ*, v. 348, g3725, Jun. 2014. DOI: 10.1136/bmj.g3725.
ILLICH, Ivan. *Medical Nemesis: The Expropriation of Health*. London: Calder & Boyars, 1975.
IOANNIDIS, John P. A. Why most published research findings are false. *PLoS Medicine*, v. 2, n. 8, p. e124, Aug. 2005. DOI: 10.1371/journal.pmed.0020124.

KROGSBØLL, Lasse T. et al. General health checks in adults for reducing morbidity and mortality from disease. *Cochrane Database of Systematic Reviews*, n. 1, CD009009, Jan. 2019. DOI: 10.1002/14651858.CD009009.pub3.

LISS, D. T. et al. General Health Checks in Adult Primary Care: A Review. *JAMA*, v. 325, n. 22, p. 2294-2306, 8 Jun. 2021.

WORLD HEALTH ORGANIZATION. *Closing the gap in a generation: health equity through action on the social determinants of health*. Geneva: WHO, 2008.

REISER, Stanley Joel. *Technological medicine: the changing world of doctors and patients*. New York: Cambridge University Press, 2009.

ROSE, Nikolas. *The Politics of Life Itself: Biomedicine, Power, and Subjectivity in the Twenty-First Century*. Princeton: Princeton University Press, 2007.

ROSENBERG, Charles E. *The Care of Strangers: The Rise of America's Hospital System*. New York: Basic Books, 1987.

SNOW K, GALAVIZ K, TURBOW. Patient Outcomes Following Interhospital Care Fragmentation: A Systematic Review. *J Gen Intern Med*. 2020;35(4):1550-1558. doi:10.1007/s11606-019-05366-z.

TOPOL, Eric. *Deep Medicine: How Artificial Intelligence Can Make Healthcare Human Again*. New York: Basic Books, 2019.

TSAO CW, Aday AW, Almarzooq ZI, et al. Heart Disease and Stroke Statistics-2022 Update: A Report From the American Heart Association. 2022;145(8):e153-e639. doi:10.1161/CIR.0000000000001052

VESALIUS, Andreas. *De Humani Corporis Fabrica Libri Septem*. Basel: Ex officina Ioannis Oporini, 1543.

WELCH, H. Gilbert; SCHWARTZ, Lisa; WOLOSHIN, Steven. *Overdiagnosed: Making People Sick in the Pursuit of Health*. Boston: Beacon Press, 2011.

ZEEVI, David et al. Personalized Nutrition by Prediction of Glycemic Responses. *Cell*, v. 163, n. 5, p. 1079-1094, Nov. 2015. DOI: 10.1016/j.cell.2015.11.001.

CHAPTER 3

AHA (Market Scan, 16 Jul 2024). Physician Burnout Rate Drops, but Still Exceeds 50%. Available at: https://www.aha.org/aha-center-health-innovation-market-scan/2024-07-16-work-remains-physician-burnout-rates-are-coming-down

BRAZILIAN MEDICAL ASSOCIATION; SÃO PAULO MEDICAL ASSOCIATION. *Unprecedented survey: doctors and the Covid-19 pandemic*. São Paulo: AMB, Jan. 2021. Available at: https://amb.org.br/noticias/pesquisa-inedita-os-medicos-e-a-pandemia-de-covid-19/

CANADIAN MEDICAL ASSOCIATION. *Physician burnout in Canada: A national survey*. Ottawa: CMA, 2022. Available at: https://www.cma.ca/sites/default/files/2022-08/NPHS_final_report_EN.pdf

BRAZIL. Ministry of Health. *Conecte SUS: National Digital Health Platform*. Brasília: Ministry of Health, 2023. Available at: https://www.gov.br/saude

DELTA BOTS. *Health innovation solutions for municipalities and clinics*. Pitangui (MG): Delta Bots, 2023. Available at: https://delta-bots-pit.webnode.page/

EPIC SYSTEMS CORPORATION. *About Epic*. Verona (WI): Epic Systems, 2023. Institutional page. Available at: https://www.epic.com

GALVÃO, A. P. F. C., SOARES, S. M., AGUIAR, F. O. de, MARQUES, L. M., OTANI, V. H. O., & UCHIDA, R. R. (2025). Detection of Anxiety in university students through voice acoustics from audios in WhatsApp Chatbot: a machine learning study. *Scire Salutis*, 15(2), e8700. https://doi.org/10.6008/CBPC2236-9600.2025.002.0010

GOOGLE HEALTH. *Med-PaLM: Large language models in medical QA*. Mountain View: Google Research, 2023. Institutional page. Available at: https://health.google

GREENHALGH, T. et al. Evidence based medicine: a movement in crisis? *BMJ*, 2014; 348:g3725 doi:10.1136/bmj.g3725

HOLLAND, J. H. *Hidden order: how adaptation builds complexity*. Reading, MA: Addison-Wesley, 1995.

HOSPITALES DIGITALES. *Public health computerization program*. Santiago: Ministry of Health of Chile, 2020. Available at: https://www.youtube.com/HospitalDigital Chile

INOVA HC - HOSPITAL DAS CLÍNICAS DA USP. *Interoperability in Health: from concept to practice at InovaHC*. São Paulo: HCFMUSP, 2022. Available at: https://inovahc.com.br/interoperabilidade-na-saude-do-conceito-a-pratica-no-inovahc/

INSTITUTE FOR HEALTHCARE IMPROVEMENT. Boston: IHI, 2021. Available at: https://www.ihi.org

IORA HEALTH. [Acquired by Amazon in 2021]. Available at: https://www.healthcaredive.com/news/amazon-one-medical-seniors-iora-rebrand/696157/

JOINT COMMISSION. *Sentinel Event Data Root Causes by Event Type: 2017 Annual Report*. Oakbrook Terrace: JC, 2017. Available at: https://www.jointcommission.org

KAUSHIK & SHARMA. Addison's disease presenting as depression. *Indian J Med Sci*, PUBMED, 2003;57(6):249-251.

KRY INTERNATIONAL. Stockholm: Kry, 2023. Institutional page. Available at: https://www.kry.se

LIVO HEALTH. *Digital transformation in clinical nursing*. Madrid: Livo, 2023. Available at: https://getlivo.com/

MAYO CLINIC CENTER FOR INNOVATION. *Time-use studies among physicians*. Rochester: Mayo Clinic, 2017. Available at: https://www.mayo.edu

MEDSCAPE. *2023 Physician Compensation Report*. New York: WebMD, 2023. Available at: https://www.medscape.com/slideshow/2023-compensation-overview-6016167

MORIN, E. *Seven Complex Lessons in Education for the Future*. 23rd ed. Rio de Janeiro: Bertrand Brasil, 2020.

MOUNT SINAI HEALTH SYSTEM. Mount Sinai to implement Dragon Copilot for clinical documentation. *YahooNews*, November/2025. Available at: https://www.yahoo.com/news/articles/mount-sinai-implement-dragon-copilot-143118223.html

NHS. *The General Practice Forward View*. London: NHS, 2016. Available at: https://www.england.nhs.uk/publication/general-practice-forward-view-gpfv/

NHS. *Paper-free at the Point of Care*. London: NHS, 2016. Available at: https://digital.nhs.uk

NOTABLE HEALTH. *AI to reduce administrative burden on doctors*. San Francisco: Notable, 2023. Available at: https://www.notablehealth.com

OPENNOTES. *Movement for transparent medical records*. Boston: Beth Israel Deaconess Medical Center, 2023. Available at: https://www.opennotes.org

PARDINI TECH. *Clinical and laboratory data intelligence*. Belo Horizonte: Pardini Group, 2023. Available at: https://www.grupopardini.com.br/

PERU. Ministry of Health. *Integrated Health System – History and challenges*. Lima: MINSA, 2022. Available at: https://www.gob.pe/minsa

SCHÖN, D. A. *The reflective practitioner: how professionals think in action*. New York: Basic Books, 1983.

SNOW K. et al., Patient Outcomes Following Interhospital Care Fragmentation: A Systematic Review, *JGIM* 2020;35(5):1550-1558; doi:10.1007/s11606-019-05366-z

TAI-SEALE, M. et al. Listening time during medical encounters: a cross-sectional study. *Mayo Clinic Proceedings*, Rochester, v. 92, n. 9, p. 1316–1324, 2017. DOI: 10.1016/j.-mayocp.2017.06.004.

TOPOL, E.J. High-performance medicine: the convergence of human and artificial intelligence. *Nat Med* 25, 44–56 (2019). https://doi.org/10.1038/s41591-018-0300-7

SINGH H et al. Types and origins of diagnostic errors in primary care settings. *JAMA Intern Med*. 2013;173(6):418-425. doi:10.1001/jamainternmed.2013.2777

SUKI AI. *Clinical documentation by voice command*. Redwood City: Suki Inc., 2023. Available at: https://www.suki.ai

STANFORD MEDICINE. *Integrated multidisciplinary team models*. Stanford: School of Medicine, 2023. Available at: https://med.stanford.edu

TAI-SEALE M, OLSON CW, LI J, et al. Electronic Health Record Logs Indicate That Physicians Split Time Evenly Between Seeing Patients And Desktop Medicine. *Health Aff (Millwood)*. PUBMED. 2017;36(4):655-662. doi:10.1377/hlthaff.2016.0811

VAN DER LEI, J. Use and abuse of computer-stored medical records. *Methods of Information in Medicine*, v. 30, n. 2, p. 79–80, 1991.

YAMAGUCHI, Ren. Japan's AI-Powered Healthcare: Transforming Patient Care. *IT Business Today*, 6 May 2025. Available at: https://itbusinesstoday.com/tech/japans-ai-powered-healthcare-transforming-patient-care/

CHAPTER 4

AUSTIN E, et al. Use of patient-generated health data across healthcare settings: implications for health systems. *JAMIA Open*. 2020;3(1):70-76. doi:10.1093/jamiaopen/ooz065.

BEIDELSCHIES M, et al. Association of the Functional Medicine Model of Care With Patient-Reported Health-Related Quality-of-Life Outcomes. *JAMA Network Open*. 2019;2(10):e1914017. doi:10.1001/jamanetworkopen.2019.14017

GRABER ML, Franklin N, Gordon R. Diagnostic Error in Internal Medicine. *Arch Intern Med*. 2005;165(13):1493–1499. doi:10.1001/archinte.165.13.1493

GREENHALGH T, Heath I. *Measuring Quality in the Therapeutic Relationship*. The King's Fund GP Inquiry; 2010 (report).

LUPTON, Deborah. *Digital Sociology*. London: Routledge, 2015.

MOL, Annemarie. *The Body Multiple: Ontology in Medical Practice*. Durham: Duke University Press, 2002.

OFRI, Danielle. *What Patients Say, What Doctors Hear*. Boston: Beacon Press, 2017.

SCHIFF GD, et al. Diagnostic Error in Medicine: Analysis of 583 Physician-Reported

Errors. *Arch Intern Med.* 2009;169(20):1881-1887. doi:10.1001/archinternmed.2009.333

TINETTI ME, Esterson J, et al. Patient Priority-Directed Decision Making and Care for Older Adults with Multiple Chronic Conditions. *Clin Geriatr Med.* 2016;32(2):261-275. doi:10.1016/j.cger.2016.01.012.

CHAPTER 5

NATIONAL SUPPLEMENTAL HEALTH AGENCY (ANS). *Sector Data and Indicators.* Rio de Janeiro: ANS, 2025. Available at: https://www.gov.br/ans/pt-br/acesso-a-informacao/perfil-do-setor/dados-e-indicadores-do-setor

Ministry of Health. *National Health Promotion Policy: PNPS – Annex I of Consolidation Ordinance No. 2, of September 28, 2017.* Brasília: MS; 2018. Available at: https://bvsms.saude.gov.br/bvs/publicacoes/politica_nacional_promocao_saude.pdf

BUENO B, Leo JD, Macfie H. IHI Leadership Alliance. *Trillion Dollar Checkbook": Reduce Waste and Cost in the US Health Care System.* Boston: Institute for Healthcare Improvement; 2019. Available at www.ihi.org.

COSGROVE L, Krimsky S. A Comparison of DSM-IV and DSM-5 Panel Members' Financial Associations with Industry: A Pernicious Problem Persists. *PLoS Med.* 2012;9(3):e1001190. doi:10.1371/journal.pmed.1001190.

DATASUS. *SUS Ambulatory Production.* Brasília: Ministry of Health. Available at: http://tabnet.datasus.gov.br

DIAGNOSTIC AND STATISTICAL MANUAL OF MENTAL DISORDERS (DSM-5). *Diagnostic and Statistical Manual of Mental Disorders.* 5th ed. Porto Alegre: Artmed, 2014.

FRENK, Julio, et al. Health professionals for a new century: transforming education to strengthen health systems in an interdependent world. *The Lancet*, v. 376, n. 9756, p. 1923-1958, 2010.

GAYNOR M, Ho K, Town RJ. The industrial organization of health-care markets. *Journal of Economic Literature.* 2015;53(2):235-284. doi:10.1257/jel.53.2.235.

GLOBAL WELLNESS INSTITUTE. *The Global Wellness Economy: Country Rankings.* Miami, FL: GWI, 2022. Available at: https://globalwellnessinstitute.org/industry-research/featured-reports/

GREENHALGH, Trisha; HOWICK, Jeremy; Maskrey, Nicholas. Evidence based medicine: a movement in crisis?. *BMJ* 2014;348:g3725. doi:10.1136/bmj.g3725.

ILLICH, Ivan. *Medical Nemesis: The Expropriation of Health.* 5th ed. São Paulo: Paulus, 2021. (Original publication 1975).

IOANNIDIS, John P. A. Why Most Published Research Findings Are False. *PLoS Medicine*, v. 2, n. 8, p. e124, 2005.

IQVIA. *The Global Use of Medicines 2023: Outlook to 2027.* Danbury, CT: IQVIA Institute for Human Data Science, 2023. Available at: https://www.iqvia.com/insights/the-iqvia-institute/reports/the-global-use-of-medicines-2023

LUNDH A, Lexchin J, Mintzes B, Schroll JB, Bero L. Industry sponsorship and research outcome. *Cochrane Database of Systematic Reviews.* 2017;(2):MR000033. doi:10.1002/14651858.MR000033.pub3

MCKINSEY & COMPANY. *Prioritizing health: A prescription for prosperity*. McKinsey Global Institute, 2020. [Report containing projection on chronic disease costs].

MEDPAC. *The Hospital Readmissions Reduction Program has succeeded for beneficiaries and the Medicare program* (2018). Available at https://www.medpac.gov/the-hospital-readmissions-reduction-program-has-succeeded-for-beneficiaries-and-the-medicare-program/

MONCRIEFF J, Cooper RE, Stockmann T, et al. The serotonin theory of depression: a systematic umbrella review of the evidence. *Molecular Psychiatry*. 2023;28:3243-3256. doi:10.1038/s41380-022-01661-0.

PURDUE PHARMA. *Justice Department Announces Global Resolution of Criminal and Civil Investigations with Opioid Manufacturer Purdue Pharma and Shareholder Members of the Sackler Family*. Washington, D.C.: U.S. Department of Justice, 2020. Available at: https://www.justice.gov/opa/pr/justice-department-announces-global-resolution-criminal-and-civil-investigations-opioid

SARPATWARI A, Sinha MS, Kesselheim AS. The Opioid Epidemic: Fixing a Broken Pharmaceutical Market. *Harvard Law & Policy Review*. 2017.

WHELTON PK, Carey RM, Aronow WS, et al. Guideline for the Prevention, Detection, Evaluation, and Management of High Blood Pressure in Adults. *ACC/AHA*. 2018;71(19):e127-e248. doi:10.1016/j.jacc.2017.11.006.

CHAPTER 6

AMERICAN BOARD OF INTERNAL MEDICINE FOUNDATION. *Choosing Wisely*. Philadelphia: ABIM Foundation, 2012–2025. Available at: https://www.-choosingwisely.org

BARSKY, Arthur J. *Worried Sick: Our Troubled Quest for Wellness*. New York: Little, Brown and Company, 2008.

BIOSALUD DAY HOSPITAL. *Regenerative medicine*. Zaragoza, ESP. Available at: https://www.biosalud.org

BRAZIL. Ministry of Health. Secretariat of Primary Health Care. *Guidelines for the Prevention of Chronic Diseases in Primary Health Care*. Brasília: Ministry of Health, 2020.

LI, L.; WANG, Y.; ZHANG, Y. et al. Analysis of the status and influencing factors of physical examination behavior among residents in China. *Chinese Journal of Preventive Medicine*, v. 55, n. 4, p. 385-390, 2021. PMID: 33847715.

CLINIQUE LA PRAIRIE. *Longevity and Wellness Clinic*. Montreux: CLP, [n.d.]. Available at: https://www.cliniquelaprairie.com.

GINGER (now Headspace). *Mental Health Care for Employees*. Available at: https://www.headspace.com/work

GRAND VIEW RESEARCH. *Corporate Wellness Market Size, Share & Trends Analysis Report — Brazil, 2024-2030*. San Francisco: GVR, 2025. Available at: https://www.grandviewresearch.com/horizon/outlook/corporate-wellness-market/brazil.

KLINIK ST. GEORG. *Specialized Clinic in Internal Medicine*. Bad Aibling, DEU. Available at: https://www.klinik-st-georg.de

KROGSBØLL, Lasse T.; JØRGENSEN, Karsten J.; GØTZSCHE, Peter C. General health checks in adults for reducing morbidity and mortality from disease. *Cochrane*

Database of Systematic Reviews. 2019;(1):CD009009. doi: 10.1002/14651858.CD009009.pub3.

LAURA. *Artificial Intelligence for Health.* Curitiba, BRA. Available at: https://lauranetworks.com/conheca-o-robo-laura/

MOLD, James W.; UNCLE, Dennis. The periodic health examination: a relic of the past? *BMJ Quality & Safety*, v. 23, n. 11, p. 882-884, 2014. doi: 10.1136/bmjqs-2014-003194.

NEXT HEALTH. *Health and Longevity Optimization Centers.* Los Angeles, USA. Available at: https://www.next-health.com

NODA, Shingo et al. Association between regular health check-ups and subsequent medical costs in a Japanese population: a retrospective cohort study. *Journal of General Internal Medicine*, v. 36, n. 11, p. 3369-3375, 2021. doi: 10.1007/s11606-021-06734-2.

PARACELSUS KLINIK LUSTMÜHLE. *Biological Medicine Center.* Lustmühle, SUI. Available at: https://www.paracelsus.ch

PING AN GOOD DOCTOR. *Health Services Platform.* Shanghai, CHN. Available at: https://www.pagd.net

PROCHAZKA AV; Caverly T. General Health Checks in Adults for Reducing Morbidity and Mortality From Disease. *JAMA.* 2019;321(24):2423-2424. doi: 10.1001/jama.2019.7844.

SCHWARTZ AL et al. Measuring Low-Value Care in Medicare. *JAMA Intern Med.* 2014;174(7):1067-1076. doi: 10.1001/jamainternmed.2014.1541.

SOUTH AFRICAN MEDICAL JOURNAL. ROTHBERG, A. D.; BERGER, D. Are annual medical check-ups worthwhile? A review of the evidence. *South African Medical Journal*, v. 107, n. 9, p. 741-743, 2017.

THE CENTER FOR INNOVATIVE MEDICINE. Johns Hopkins Medicine. Baltimore, USA. Available at: https://www.hopkinsmedicine.org/innovative-medicine

U.S. PREVENTIVE SERVICES TASK FORCE (USPSTF). *Clinical Guidelines and Recommendations.* Available at: https://www.uspreventiveservicestaskforce.org

CHAPTER 7

ADA HEALTH. Institutional Page. Berlin, Germany. Available at: https://ada.com

ADELI, K.; HIGGINS, V.; TRAJCEVSKI, K.; WHITE-Al HABEEB, N. The Canadian Laboratory Initiative on Pediatric Reference Intervals: White Paper CALIPER. *Critical Reviews in Clinical Laboratory Sciences*, 54(6):358–413, 2017. doi:10.1080/10408363.2017.1379945.

AMERICAN COLLEGE OF CARDIOLOGY (ACC). Institutional Page. Washington, D.C., USA. Available at: https://www.acc.org.

BALOGH, Erin P.; MILLER, Bryan T.; BALL, John R. (Eds.). *Improving Diagnosis in Health Care.* Washington (DC): National Academies Press (US), 2015.

BEARABLE. *Symptom & Mood Tracker App.* London, GBR. Available at: https://bearable.app/

CARA CARE. *Digital therapeutics for digestive health.* Berlin, DEU. Available at: https://cara.care/

CAREvolution. *Development of innovative services to improve health and well-being.* [European Startup]. Available at: https://www.carevolution.be/

CLEVELAND CLINIC CENTER FOR FUNCTIONAL MEDICINE. Institutional Page. Cleveland, USA. Available at: https://my.clevelandclinic.org/departments/functional-medicine

DIABETES PREVENTION PROGRAM RESEARCH GROUP. Reduction in the incidence of type 2 diabetes with lifestyle intervention or metformin. *The New England Journal of Medicine*, v. 346, n. 6, p. 393-403, 2002.

DUTCH TEST (Precision Analytical). *Hormone tests.* McMinnville, USA. Available at: https://dutchtest.com

ELLIPSIS HEALTH. *AI voice biomarker for behavioral health.* Available at: https://www.ellipsishealth.com

ENDOCRINE SOCIETY. Institutional Page. Washington, D.C., USA. Available at: https://www.endocrine.org

FUNCTIONAL MIND. *AI Operating System for Functional Medicine.* Available at: https://functionalmind.ai/

GLEICHER, Norbert, et al. Misleading and deceptive advertising in reproductive medicine. *Fertility and Sterility*, v. 116, n. 4, p. 936-940, 2021.

HEARTMATH INSTITUTE. Institutional Page. Boulder Creek, USA. Available at: https://www.heartmath.org

INSIDE TRACKER. *Personalized health analysis.* Cambridge, USA. Available at: https://www.insidetracker.com

INSTITUTE FOR FUNCTIONAL MEDICINE (IFM). Institutional Page. Federal Way, USA. Available at: https://www.ifm.org

OMNILAMP. *Portable molecular diagnostics.* [Brazilian startup]. FAPEMIG, 2023. Available at: http://www.fapemig.br/pt/noticias/932/

ROSE, Geoffrey. *The Strategy of Preventive Medicine.* Oxford: Oxford University Press, 1992.

SARRIS, J., et al. Nutritional medicine as mainstream in psychiatry. *The Lancet Psychiatry*, v. 2, n. 3, p. 271-274, 2015.

TALIAZ. *AI-empowered mental health.* Tel Aviv, ISR. Available at: https://www.taliazhealth.com

VAUCHER, P. et al. Effect of iron supplementation on fatigue in nonanemic menstruating women with low ferritin: a randomized controlled trial. *CMAJ*, 184(11):1247-1254, 2012. doi:10.1503/cmaj.110950.

VERNON, G.; BARANOVA, A.; YOUNOSSI, Z.M. Systematic review: the epidemiology and natural history of non-alcoholic fatty liver disease and non-alcoholic steatohepatitis in adults. *Alimentary Pharmacology & Therapeutics*, 34(3):274–285, 2011. doi:10.1111/j.1365-2036.2011.04724.x.

YAZDANI S, Hosseinzadeh M, Hosseini F. Models of clinical reasoning with a focus on general practice: A critical review. *J Adv Med Educ Prof.* 2017;5(4):177-184.

ZHANG, Lihua, et al. Long-Term Cumulative High-Sensitivity C-Reactive Protein and Mortality Among Patients With Acute Heart Failure. *Journal of the American Heart Association*, v. 12, n. 19, p. e031572, Oct. 2023. DOI: 10.1161/JAHA.123.031572.

CHAPTER 8

ABRIDGE. *Medical consultation listening with generative AI technology*. Available at: https://www.abridge.com

AMERICAN MEDICAL ASSOCIATION (AMA). *Physician Burnout*. Available at: https://amaalliance.org/physician-burnout/

ARNDT, B.G. et al. Tethered to the EHR: Primary Care Physician Workload Assessment Using EHR Event Log Data and Time-Motion Observations. *Annals of Family Medicine*, 15(5):419–426, 2017. PMID: 28893811.

NATIONAL ASSOCIATION OF OCCUPATIONAL MEDICINE (ANMT). *Information Bulletin on Mental Health and Work*. Brasília: ANMT. [Data on burnout in Brazil]. Available at: https://www.anamt.org.br

SÃO PAULO MEDICAL ASSOCIATION (APM). *Survey on Physicians' Working Conditions in São Paulo during the COVID-19 pandemic*. São Paulo: APM, June 2020. Available at: https://www.apm.org.br/wp-content/uploads/10_jun2020_Pesquisa-APM_medicos-e-covid19_03.pdf

CANADIAN MEDICAL ASSOCIATION (CMA). *The 2021 National Physician Health Survey*. Ottawa: CMA, 2021. Available at: https://www.cma.ca/physician-wellness-hub/resources/national-physician-health-survey-reports

CLINICAL PATHWAYS. *Visual tool for clinical decision support*. London, UK. Available at: https://clinicalpathways.uk/

FEDERAL COUNCIL OF MEDICINE (CFM). *Reports and Resolutions on Medical Practice and Health Systems*. Brasília: CFM. Available at: https://portal.cfm.org.br

COIMBRA, B.M. et al. Moral injury and mental health among health-care workers during the COVID-19 pandemic: a systematic review and meta-analysis. *Journal of Affective Disorders*, 2023/2024. PMCID: PMC10776063.

DELTA BOTS. *AI and Automation Solutions for Health*. Pitangui, BRA. Available at: https://delta-bots-pit.webnode.page/sobre-nos/

EPIC SYSTEMS. *Electronic Health Records*. Verona, USA. Available at: https://www.epic.com

FABICHAK C, SILVA-JUNIOR, J; MORRONE, L. C. Burnout Syndrome in medical residents and organizational work predictors. *Revista Brasileira de Medicina do Trabalho*. 2014;12(2) DOI::79-84.

GAWANDE, Atul. Why Doctors Hate Their Computers. *The New Yorker*, 12 Nov. 2018.

GÓMEZ-URQUIZA, José L.; VARGAS-CIÁRRAGA, Raquel E.; GONZÁLEZ-LÓPEZ, Jesús R.; FERNÁNDEZ-CASTRO, José; DE-LA-FUENTE-SOLANA, Emilia I. Prevalence of compassion fatigue in health professionals: a systematic review and meta-analysis. *Psicodebate: Psychology, Culture and Society*, v. 17, n. 1, p. 89-101, 2017.

HOSPITAL DAS CLÍNICAS (FMUSP). *Innovation and Interoperability Projects in Health*. São Paulo, BRA. Available at: https://inovahc.hc.fm.usp.br/quem-somos/

IORA HEALTH (now part of One Medical). *Primary Care Model*. Available at: https://www.onemedical.com

JOINT COMMISSION, The. *Sentinel Event Alert 57: The essential role of leadership in developing a safety culture*. Oakbrook Terrace, IL, 2017.

KING'S FUND, The. *The courage of compassion: Supporting nurses and midwives to deliver high-quality care*. London: The King's Fund, 2020. Available at: https://www.kingsfund.org.uk/insight-and-analysis/reports/courage-compassion-supporting-nurses-midwives

KRY (LIVI). *Digital Healthcare Provider*. Stockholm, SWE. Available at: https://www.kry.se

LIVO. *Nursing Roster Management Platform*. Barcelona, ESP. Available at: https://getlivo.com/

MARBURGER BUND. *Doctors' Union of Germany*. Berlin, DEU. Available at: https://www.marburger-bund.de

MEDSCAPE. *Physician Burnout & Depression Report 2023: 'I Cry but No One Cares'*: Medscape, 2023.

MEU SUS DIGITAL (Conecte SUS). *Brazilian Citizen's Official Health Platform*. Brasília: Ministry of Health. Available at: https://meususdigital.saude.gov.br

MY HEALTH RECORD. *Australia's National Digital Health System*. Sydney, AUS. Available at: https://www.myhealthrecord.gov.au

NATIONAL HEALTH SERVICE (NHS). *The Paperless 2020 programme*. London, UK. [Government program].

NOTABLE. *Intelligent Automation for Healthcare*. Available at: https://www.notablehealth.com

OPENNOTES. *A movement to make health care more open and transparent*. Boston: Beth Israel Deaconess Medical Center. Available at: https://www.opennotes.org

WORLD HEALTH ORGANIZATION (WHO). *Healthy workplaces: a global model for action*. Geneva: WHO, 2010.

PANAGIOTI M, Geraghty K, Johnson J, et al. Association Between Physician Burnout and Patient Safety, Professionalism, and Patient Satisfaction: A Systematic Review and Meta-analysis. *JAMA Intern Med*. 2018;178(10):1317–1331. doi:10.1001/jamainternmed.2018.3713

PHELCOM. *Technology and Innovation in Ophthalmology*. São Carlos, BRA. Available at: https://phelcom.com.br

SCHÖN, Donald A. *The Reflective Practitioner: How Professionals Think in Action*. New York: Basic Books, 1983.

STANFORD MEDICINE WELLMD & WELLPHD CENTER. Stanford, USA. Available at: https://wellmd.stanford.edu

SUKI AI. *Voice solutions with AI technology for healthcare*. Redwood City, USA. Available at: https://www.suki.ai

CHAPTER 9

ALFRADIQUE, M. E., et al. Hospitalizations for ambulatory care sensitive conditions: the construction of the Brazilian list as a tool for measuring health system performance (Project ICSAP – Brazil). *Cadernos de Saúde Pública*, v. 25, n. 6, p. 1337-1349, 2009.

AMERICAN BOARD OF INTERNAL MEDICINE (ABIM) FOUNDATION. *Choosing Wisely*. Available at: https://www.choosingwisely.org

AMERICAN HEART ASSOCIATION (AHA). *Heart Attack Symptoms in Women*. Dallas, USA: AHA, 2022. [Statement regarding the cited warning]. Available at:

https://www.heart.org/en/health-topics/heart-attack/warning-signs-of-a-heart-attack/heart-attack-symptoms-in-women

COLUMBIA UNIVERSITY. *Division of Narrative Medicine.* Available at: https://www.narrativemedicine.org

FOOD AND DRUG ADMINISTRATION (FDA). *2023 Drug Trials Snapshots Summary Report.* Silver Spring, MD: U.S. Department of Health and Human Services, 2024. Available at: https://www.fda.gov/drugs/drug-approvals-and-databases/drug-trials-snapshots

GREEN, M. L. Evidence-based medicine training in internal medicine residency programs: a national survey. *Journal of General Internal Medicine*, v. 15, n. 2, p. 129-133, 2000. doi:10.1046/j.1525-1497.2000.03379.x.

HARVARD MEDICAL SCHOOL. *Center for Bioethics: Medical Humanities.* [Initiative representative of narrative medicine teaching]. Available at: https://bioethics.hms.harvard.edu/

LUNDH, Andreas, et al. Industry sponsorship and research outcome. *Cochrane Database of Systematic Reviews*, n. 2, 2017.

MOL, Annemarie. *The Logic of Care: Health and the Problem of Patient Choice.* London: Routledge, 2008.

WORLD HEALTH ORGANIZATION (WHO). *Framework for evidence-informed policy-making.* Geneva: WHO, 2021.

REALISTIC MEDICINE. *Chief Medical Officer for Scotland's Annual Report.* Edinburgh: The Scottish Government. [Government initiative]. Available at: https://www.gov.scot/publications/chief-medical-officers-annual-report-2024-2025-realistic-medicine-critical-connections/

ROYAL COLLEGE OF GENERAL PRACTITIONERS (RCGP). *Fit for the Future: A vision for general practice.* London: RCGP, 2019.

SCHRIJVER, Iris; BRADY, Keri J. S.; TROCKEL, Mickey. An exploration of key issues and potential solutions that impact physician wellbeing and professional fulfillment at an academic center. *PeerJ*, [S. l.], v. 4, e1853, 10 Mar. 2016. Available at: https://peerj.com/articles/1783/

STENGERS, Isabelle. *Another Science is Possible: A Manifesto for Slow Science.* Paris: La Découverte, 2013.

TOPOL, Eric. *Deep Medicine: How Artificial Intelligence Can Make Healthcare Human Again.* New York: Basic Books, 2019.

VYAS, Darshali A.; EISENSTEIN, Leo G.; JONES, David S. Hidden in Plain Sight — Reconsidering the Use of Race Correction in Clinical Algorithms. *The New England Journal of Medicine*, v. 383, n. 9, p. 874-882, 2020.

CHAPTER 10

AFFECTIVA. *AI to capture and detect complex human cognitive and emotional states.* Institutional page. Boston, USA. Available at: https://www.affectiva.com

ALAM, Mohammad Arif Ul et al. AutoCogniSys: IoT Assisted Context-Aware Automatic Cognitive Health Assessment. In: *EAI International Conference on Mobile and Ubiquitous Systems: Computing, Networking and Services.* New York: ACM, August 2021. p. 184-195. Available at: https://doi.org/10.1145/3448891.3448945

ALLIANCE FOR HEALTHIER COMMUNITIES. *Rx: Community — Social Prescribing in Ontario*. Available at: https://www.allianceon.org/Rx-Community-Social-Prescribing-In-Ontario

AMERICAN COLLEGE OF LIFESTYLE MEDICINE. *Lifestyle Medicine Residency Curriculum*. Available at: https://lifestylemedicine.org/project/residency-curriculum/

BARSKY, Arthur J, BORUS J.F. Functional somatic syndromes. *Annals of Internal Medicine*. 1999;130:910-921. Vol. 130, N. 11. doi:10.7326/0003-4819-130-11-199906010-00016

BIOBEAT. *Remote monitoring of patients with hypertension*. Institutional page. Available at: https://www.bio-beat.com/

CIRCLE OF SECURITY INTERNATIONAL. *Relationship-based early intervention program*. Institutional page. Available at: https://www.circleofsecurityinternational.com

COLE, S. W. Human Social Genomics. *PLoS Genetics*, v. 10, n. 8, e1004601, 2014. doi:10.1371/journal.pgen.1004601

DANA-FARBER CANCER INSTITUTE. *Psychosocial Oncology and Palliative Care*. Boston, USA. Institutional page. Available at: https://www.dana-farber.org/

DANNER, D. D., SNOWDON, D. A., & FRIESEN, W. V. (2001). Positive emotions in early life and longevity: Findings from the nun study. *Journal of Personality and Social Psychology*, 80(5), 804–813. https://doi.org/10.1037/0022-3514.80.5.804

EDWARDS RR, DWORKIN RH, SULLIVAN MD, TURK DC, WASAN AD. The Role of Psychosocial Processes in the Development and Maintenance of Chronic Pain. *J Pain*. 2016;17(9 Suppl):T70-T92. doi:10.1016/j.jpain.2016.01.001

ELLIPSIS HEALTH. *AI voice biomarker for behavioral health*. Institutional page. Available at: https://www.ellipsishealth.com

EMPATICA. *Platform with AI technology for health monitoring*. Institutional page. Available at: https://www.empatica.com

EMTEQ. *Facial expression detection technology and biometrics*. Institutional page. Available at: https://www.emteqlabs.com

FEEL THERAPEUTICS. *Wearable and AI app, precision medicine for mental health*. Institutional page. Available at: https://www.feeltherapeutics.com/

FIELD, L. H.; EDWARDS, S. D.; EDWARDS, D. J.; DEAN, S. E. Influence of HeartMath Training Programme on Physiological and Psychological Variables. *Global Journal of Health Science*, v. 10, n. 2, p. 126–133, 2018. doi:10.5539/gjhs.v10n2p126

HARVARD SCHOOL OF PUBLIC HEALTH. *The Nutrition Source*. [Representative initiative on the impact of habits]. Available at: https://www.hsph.harvard.edu/nutri tionsource/

HOLT-LUNSTAD, J.; SMITH, T. B.; LAYTON, J. B. Social Relationships and Mortality Risk: A Meta-analytic Review. *PLoS Medicine*, v. 7, n. 7, e1000316, 2010. doi:10.1371/journal.pmed.1000316.

HOSPITAIS SAUDÁVEIS. *Coalition of health institutions*. São Paulo, BRA. Available at: https://www.hospitaissaudaveis.org/

KELLY Jr., J. H.; KAHLEOVA, H.; BARNARD, N. D. The Role of Lifestyle Medicine in the Pillars of Health. *American Journal of Lifestyle Medicine*, v. 14, n. 4, p. 402–404, 2020. doi:10.1177/1559827620930971.

KYOTO UNIVERSITY HOSPITAL. Institutional page. Available at: https://www.h.kpu-m.ac.jp/en/departments/clinical-departments/psychiatry.html. Kyoto, Japan.

MATO GROSSO DO SUL. State Secretariat of Social Assistance and Human Rights. *Cuidar de Quem Cuida Program*. Available at: https://www.sead.ms.gov.br/programa-cuidar-de-quem-cuida/

MAYO CLINIC. *Health and Wellness Coaching Program*. Institutional page. Available at: https://www.mayoclinic.org/vid-20522993

MUSE. *Headband with brain sensors*. Institutional page. Available at: https://choosemuse.com

WORLD HEALTH ORGANIZATION (WHO). *Mental health and substance use*. Geneva: WHO, 2022. Available at: https://www.who.int/teams/mental-health-and-substance-use/overview

OURA. *Ring with AI for health monitoring*. Institutional page. Available at: https://ouraring.com

PONTIFICAL CATHOLIC UNIVERSITY OF RIO DE JANEIRO (PUC-Rio). *Software Engineering Laboratory (LES)*. [AI and mental health research initiative]. Rio de Janeiro, BRA. Institutional page. Available at: https://www.les.inf.puc-rio.br/

SLAVICH, G. M.; IRWIN, M. R. From Stress to Inflammation and Major Depressive Disorder: A Social Signal Transduction Theory of Depression. *Psychological Bulletin*, v. 140, n. 3, p. 774–815, 2014. doi:10.1037/a0035302.

SOCIAL PRESCRIBING NETWORK (UK). *Personalized medicine initiative of the NHS - UK public health to know diverse needs affecting health*. Institutional page. Available at: https://www.england.nhs.uk/personalisedcare/social-prescribing/

SONE, T. et al. Sense of Life Worth Living (Ikigai) and Mortality in Japan: Ohsaki Study. *Psychosomatic Medicine*, v. 70, n. 6, p. 709–715, 2008.

SPIEGEL, David, et al. Effect of psychosocial treatment on survival of patients with metastatic breast cancer. *The Lancet*, v. 334, n. 8668, p. 888-891, 1989. [Seminal study that inspired the Social Support Intervention Trial].

TIGNUM. *Platform focused on human performance science with personalized strategies*. Institutional page. Available at: https://www.tignum.com/solutions

UCHINO, Bert N. Social support and physical health: the behavioral pathways. *Perspectives on Psychological Science*, v. 1, n. 2, p. 74-79, 2006. doi:10.1111/j.1745-6916.2006.00012.x.

EISENDRATH SJ, Gillung E, Delucchi KL, et al. A Randomized Controlled Trial of Mindfulness-Based Cognitive Therapy for Treatment-Resistant Depression. *Psychother Psychosom*. 2016;85(2):99-110. doi:10.1159/000442260

WELLTORY. *Heart Rate Variability (HRV) and Stress Monitoring App*. Institutional page. Available at: https://welltory.com

WEN, B. et al. Health Guardian Platform: A Technology Stack to Accelerate Discovery in Digital Health Research. *arXiv*, 2022. Available at: https://arxiv.org/abs/2211.06330.

WHOOP. *Smartwatch for health and fitness*. Institutional page. Available at: https://www.whoop.com

YUSUF, Salim, et al. Effect of potentially modifiable risk factors associated with myocardial infarction in 52 countries (the INTERHEART study): case-control study. *The Lancet*, v. 364, n. 9438, p. 937-952, 2004. doi:10.1016/S0140-6736(04)17018-9.

CHAPTER 11

AL KHATIB, I. et al. A systematic review of the impact of therapeutical biophilic design on health and wellbeing of patients and care providers in healthcare services settings. *Sec. Sustainable Design and Construction*. Volume 10 - 2024. https://doi.org/10.3389/fbuil.2024.1467692.

ANDRADE, K. P.; OLIVEIRA, L. L. A.; SOUZA, R. P.; MATOS, I. M. Measurement of hospital noise level and its effects on employees based on complaint reports. *Revista CEFAC*, v. 18, n. 6, p. 1379-1388, Nov./Dec. 2016. DOI: 10.1590/1982-0216201618619815.

APARÍCIO C, Panin F. Interventions to improve inpatients' sleep quality in intensive care units and acute wards: a literature review. *Br J Nurs*. 2020;29(13):770-776. doi:10.12968/bjon.2020.29.13.770

BELTRAMI, F. G. et al.. Sleep in the intensive care unit. *Jornal Brasileiro de Pneumologia*, v. 41, n. 6, p. 539–546, Nov. 2015.

CLEVELAND CLINIC. *Integrative and Lifestyle Medicine*. Cleveland, USA. [Reference center for cited studies on sensory therapies]. Institutional page. Available at: https://my.clevelandclinic.org/departments/integrative-lifestyle-medicine

HOSPITAL DE AMOR. *Proposal of humanization and welcoming*. Institutional page. Barretos, BRA. Available at: https://hospitaldeamor.com.br/site/

HOSPITAL SÍRIO-LIBANÊS. *Integrative Care*. São Paulo, BRA. Available at: https://hospitalsiriolibanes.org.br/especialidades-medicas/sao-paulo/cuidados-integrativos/

INSTITUTE FOR PATIENT AND FAMILY-CENTERED CARE (IPFCC). Institutional Page. Bethesda, USA. Available at: https://www.ipfcc.org

KAROLINSKA INSTITUTET. *Department of Clinical Neuroscience*. Stockholm, SWE. [Reference center for research in neuroarchitecture]. Available at: https://ki.se/en/cns

KHOO TECK PUAT HOSPITAL. Singapore. Institutional page. Available at: https://www.ktph.com.sg

LAUFFENBURGER, Julie C. et al. Prescribing decision-making by medical residents on night shifts: a qualitative study. *Medical Education*, v. 56, n. 10, p. 1032–1041, Oct. 2022. DOI: 10.1111/medu.14845.

LKOUL, A.; OUMBAREK, K.; BOUCHRITI, Y.; JNIENE, A.; DENDANE, T. Environmental Factors Affecting Sleep Quality in Intensive Care Unit Patients in Southern Morocco: An Assessment Study. *Adv. Respir. Med.* 2025, 93, 14. https://doi.org/10.3390/arm93030014

MAGGIE'S CENTRE. *Support for people with cancer*. Institutional page. London, GBR. Available at: https://www.maggies.org

MASS DESIGN GROUP. *Healing Environments*. Boston, USA. Available at: https://massdesigngroup.org/design-heals-documentary

MIT Technology Review Brasil. INNOVATIVE HOSPITALS use nature for well-being. 13 Jul. 2023. Available at: https://mittechreview.com.br/hospitais-inovadores-utilizam-a-natureza-em-prol-do-bem-estar/

NÆSTVED HEALTH CENTER. Næstved, DEN. Institutional page. Available at: https://www.naestved.dk/sundhed-og-omsorg/sundhedstilbud

NATIONAL HEALTH SERVICE (NHS) ENGLAND. *Palliative and end of life care*. London, GBR. Available at: https://www.england.nhs.uk/eolc/

PAN AMERICAN HEALTH ORGANIZATION (PAHO/WHO). *Report on Quality of Care in Emergency Services in Latin America*. 2024. Available at: https://www.paho.org/pub/pt/relatorio-anual-2024/

PLUMMER, N. R. et al. SoundEar noise warning devices cause a sustained reduction in ambient sound overnight in adult critical care units. *Journal of the Intensive Care Society*, 2018.

SOUNDEAR. [Noise monitoring solutions for hospitals] Aarhus, DEN. Available at: https://soundear.com/

ULRICH, Roger S., et al. A Review of the Research Literature on Evidence-Based Healthcare Design. *Health Environments Research & Design Journal*, v. 1, n. 3, p. 61-125, 2008. doi:10.1177/193758670800100306.

ULRICH, Roger S. View through a window may influence recovery from surgery. *Science*, v. 224, n. 4647, p. 420-421, 1984. doi:10.1126/science.6143402

VAN der Schaaf PS, Dusseldorp E, Keuning FM, Janssen WA, Noorthoorn EO. Impact of the physical environment of psychiatric wards on the use of seclusion. *Br J Psychiatry*. 2013;202:142-149. doi:10.1192/bjp.bp.112.118422

WORLD HEALTH ORGANIZATION (WHO). *Environmental Noise Guidelines for the European Region*. Copenhagen: WHO Regional Office for Europe, 2018.

CHAPTER 12

AGENCY FOR HEALTHCARE RESEARCH AND QUALITY (AHRQ). *The Patient-Centered Medical Home Model*. Available at: https://www.ahrq.gov/

BRAZIL. Ministry of Health. *Family Health Strategy*. Available at: https://www.gov.br/saude/pt-br/campanhas-da-saude/2024/saude-da-familia

BRAZIL. Ministry of Health. *Better at Home Program*. Available at: https://www.gov.br/saude/pt-br/assuntos/saude-de-a-a-z/m/melhor-em-casa

BUURTZORG. Almelo, NLD. Institutional page. Available at: https://www.buurtzorg.com

CASALINO, L. P., et al. US Physician Practices Spend More Than $15.4 Billion Annually To Report Quality Measures. *Health Affairs*, v. 35, n. 3, p. 401-406, 2016. doi:10.1377/hlthaff.2015.1258.

GERBER, M. S. et al. Digital Health–Supported Lifestyle Interventions for Type 2 Diabetes: A Systematic Review and Meta-analysis of Randomized Clinical Trials. *JAMA Network Open*, v. 6, n. 7, e2333629, 2023.

INSTITUTE FOR HEALTHCARE IMPROVEMENT (IHI). *Artificial Intelligence in Health Care*. Boston: IHI. Available at: https://www.ihi.org/library/topics/artificial-intelligence

INSTITUTE OF SUPPLEMENTARY HEALTH STUDIES (IESS). *Analysis of Health Spending Profile in Brazil*. São Paulo: IESS, 2023. Available at: https://www2.iess.org.br/cms/rep/estudo_especial_gastos.pdf

INSTITUTE OF APPLIED ECONOMIC RESEARCH (IPEA). *System of Social Perception Indicators (SIPS): Health*. Brasília: IPEA, 2021. Available at: https://repositorio.ipea.gov.br/entities/book/f0e41cc8-290a-4588-8ac5-fe6b8813ffad

INSTITUTE OF MEDICINE. *Crossing the Quality Chasm: A New Health System for the*

21st Century. Washington, DC: National Academies Press, 2001. doi:10.17226/10027.
PEYROT, M. et al. Diabetes Attitudes, Wishes and Needs (DAWN): study design and methods. *Diabetic Medicine*, v. 22, n. 7, p. 943–952, 2005. doi:10.1111/j.1464-5491.2005.01544.x.
BELO HORIZONTE CITY HALL. *Home Care*. Belo Horizonte, BRA. [Municipal program]. Available at: https://prefeitura.pbh.gov.br/saude/informacoes/atencao-a-saude/urgencia-e-emergencia/servico-de-atendimento-domiciliar
UNIFIED HEALTH SYSTEM (SUS). *Brazilian Government Portal*. Brasília, BRA. Available at: https://www.gov.br/saude/pt-br/assuntos/sus
SMITH, S. M. et al. Interventions for improving outcomes in patients with multimorbidity in primary care and community settings. *BMJ*, v. 345, e5205, 2012. doi:10.1136/bmj.e5205.
SHAH, N. H.; MILSTEIN, A.; BAGLEY, S. C. Making Health Care Smarter. *JAMA*, v. 322, n. 5, p. 397–398, 2019. doi:10.1001/jama.2019.8846.
SHIELDS GS, Spahr CM, Slavich GM. Psychosocial Interventions and Immune System Function: A Systematic Review and Meta-analysis of Randomized Clinical Trials. *JAMA Psychiatry*. 2020;77(10):1031–1043. doi:10.1001/jamapsychiatry.2020.0431
TELESSAÚDERS-UFRGS. Institutional Page. Porto Alegre: UFRGS. Available at: https://www.ufrgs.br/telessauders/

CHAPTER 13

ANTONOVSKY, Aaron. *Health, Stress, and Coping: New Perspectives on Mental and Physical Well-being*. San Francisco: Jossey-Bass, 1979.
ARTS IN HEALTH AT DUKE. Institutional Page. Durham, USA: Duke University Hospital. Available at: https://www.dukehealth.org/hospitals/duke-university-hospi tal/arts-health
BLACKBURN, E.; EPEL, E. *The Telomere Effect*. Lisbon: Pergaminho (Grupo Planeta), 2017. (Original title: *The Telomere Effect*, Grand Central, 2017)
BOSTON CHILDREN'S HOSPITAL. *Creative Arts Program*. Boston, USA. Available at: https://www.childrenshospital.org/patient-resources/while-you-are-here/creative-arts/art-program
BUETTNER, Dan. *The Blue Zones: Lessons for Living Longer From the People Who've Lived the Longest*. Alfragide: Nascente, 2021. (Original title: *The Blue Zones*).
CENTERS FOR DISEASE CONTROL AND PREVENTION (CDC). *Social Determinants of Health*. Available at: https://www.cdc.gov/socialdeterminants/index.htm
DESPRET, Vinciane. *What Would Animals Say If We Asked the Right Questions?*. Paris: La Découverte, 2012.
DOIDGE, Norman. *The Brain That Changes Itself: Stories of Personal Triumph from the Frontiers of Brain Science*. 7th ed. Rio de Janeiro: Record, 2011. (Original title: *The Brain That Changes Itself*).
FRANKL, Viktor E. *Man's Search for Meaning*. 49th ed. Petrópolis: Vozes, 2021. (Original title: *Man's Search for Meaning*).
FREDRICKSON, Barbara L. The broaden-and-build theory of positive emotions. *Philo-*

sophical Transactions of the Royal Society B: Biological Sciences, v. 359, n. 1449, p. 1367-1378, 2004. doi:10.1098/rstb.2004.1512.

FREITAS, Daniel Melecchi de Oliveira; SPADONI, Viviane Souto. Is virtual reality useful for pain management in patients undergoing medical procedures? *Einstein (São Paulo)*, v. 17, n. 2, eMD4837, May 2019. https://doi.org/10.31744/einstein_journal/2019MD4837

IOANNIDIS, John P. A. Why Most Published Research Findings Are False. *PLoS Medicine*, v. 2, n. 8, p. e124, 2005.

KAUFFMAN, Stuart A. *At Home in the Universe: The Search for the Laws of Self-Organization and Complexity*. New York: Oxford University Press, 1995.

LAZAR, S. W. et al. Meditation experience is associated with increased cortical thickness. *Neuroreport*, v. 16, n. 17, p. 1893–1897, 2005. doi:10.1097/01.wnr.0000186598.66243.23.

MATÉ, Gabor. *The Myth of Normal: Trauma, Illness, and Healing in a Toxic Culture*. Lisbon: Lua de Papel, 2023. (Original title: *The Myth of Normal*).

MD ANDERSON CANCER CENTER. *Integrative Medicine Center*. Houston, USA. Available at: https://www.mdanderson.org/patients-family/diagnosis-treatment/care-centers-clinics/integrative-medicine-center.html.

NATIONAL CENTER FOR COMPLEMENTARY AND INTEGRATIVE HEALTH (NCCIH). Institutional Page. Bethesda, USA: National Institutes of Health. Available at: https://www.nccih.nih.gov

WORLD HEALTH ORGANIZATION (WHO). *Health 2020: A European policy framework and strategy for the 21st century*. Copenhagen: WHO Regional Office for Europe, 2013.

ORNISH, Dean, et al. Can lifestyle changes reverse coronary heart disease? The Lifestyle Heart Trial. *The Lancet*, v. 336, n. 8708, p. 129-133, 1990. doi:10.1016/0140-6736(90)91656-U.

PORGES, Stephen W. *The Polyvagal Theory: Neurophysiological Foundations of Emotions, Attachment, Communication, and Self-regulation*. New York: W. W. Norton & Company, 2011.

PRIGOGINE, Ilya; STENGERS, Isabelle. *Order out of Chaos: Man's New Dialogue with Nature*. 3rd ed. Brasília: Editora Universidade de Brasília, 1997. (Original title: *La Nouvelle Alliance*).

ROBERT WOOD JOHNSON FOUNDATION. *Social Determinants of Health*. Available at: https://www.rwjf.org/en/insights/our-research/topics/social-determinants-of-health.html

ROGERS, Carl R. *On Becoming a Person*. 6th ed. São Paulo: WMF Martins Fontes, 2009. (Original title: *On Becoming a Person*).

SOUTHCENTRAL FOUNDATION. *Nuka System of Care*. Anchorage, USA. Available at: https://www.southcentralfoundation.com/nuka-system-of-care/

SZYF, Moshe; MEANEY, Michael J. Epigenetics, behaviour, and health. In: *A life course approach to healthy ageing*. Oxford: Oxford University Press, 2012. https://doi.org/10.1186/1710-1492-4-1-37.

UNIVERSITY OF SYDNEY. *Poche Centre for Indigenous Health*. [Reference center for cited studies]. Sydney, AUS. Available at: https://www.sydney.edu.au/medicine-health/our-research/research-centres/poche-centre-for-indigenous-health.html.

WINNICOTT, Donald W. *Playing and Reality*. Rio de Janeiro: Imago, 1975. (Original title: *Playing and Reality*).

CHAPTER 14

AMARAL, Carlos Eduardo Menezes et al. Mental health care in Brazil: a multifaceted study in four large cities. *Cadernos de Saúde Pública*, v. 37, n. 3, 2021. DOI: 10.1590/0102-311X00043420.

BRAZIL. MINISTRY OF HEALTH. *ConecteSUS*. Available at: https://www.gov.br/saude/pt-br/assuntos/conecte-sus

FEDERAL COUNCIL OF NURSING (COFEN); OSWALDO CRUZ FOUNDATION (FIOCRUZ). *Nursing Profile in Brazil: Final Report*. Brasília: Cofen/Fiocruz, 2017. Available at: http://www.cofen.gov.br/

FEDERAL COUNCIL OF NURSING (COFEN). *Survey on working conditions of nursing professionals in the context of Covid-19 in Brazil (Fiocruz)*. Brasília: Cofen, 2021. Available at: https://www.cofen.gov.br/covid-19-estudo-avalia-condicoes-de-trabalho-na-saude/

REGIONAL COUNCIL OF PHYSICAL THERAPY AND OCCUPATIONAL THERAPY OF THE 2ND REGION (CREFITO-2). *Impact of the Medical Act Law on Physical Therapy clinical practice*. Available at: https://www.crefito2.gov.br/home/conteudo/5664

CYRULNIK, Boris. *The Ugly Ducklings*. São Paulo: Martins Fontes, 2004.

SERGIO AROUCA NATIONAL SCHOOL OF PUBLIC HEALTH (ENSP/FIOCRUZ). *The dynamics of the multiprofessional team in Primary Care: a study on the construction of therapeutic plans in four Brazilian capitals*. Rio de Janeiro: Fiocruz, 2022.

FLORIANO, Mariana. Experience report. In: GADELHA, P. (org.). *Common Clinic: essays on the power of shared care*. São Paulo: Hucitec, 2021.

OSWALDO CRUZ FOUNDATION (FIOCRUZ). *ObservaRH. Report on the performance of physical therapists and occupational therapists in the public network*. Rio de Janeiro: Fiocruz, 2021. Available at: http://www.ensp.fiocruz.br/observarh/

HOSPITAL ALBERT EINSTEIN. *Innovation and Technology*. Available at: https://www.einstein.br/estrutura/inovacao

LIMA, A. C. et al. Post-COVID-19 rehabilitation in an integrated care model: the Hospital das Clínicas experience. *Frontiers in Rehabilitation Sciences*, v. 4, 2023.

WORLD HEALTH ORGANIZATION (WHO). *State of the World's Nursing 2020: Investing in education, jobs and leadership*. Geneva: WHO, 2020.

PHILIPS. *Tasy EMR: Electronic Medical Record*. Available at: https://www.philips.com.br/healthcare/product/HC881113/tasy-emr-prontuario-eletronico-do-paciente

REEVES, S. et al. Multiprofessional teamwork in primary care: a study of barriers and facilitators. *Journal of Interprofessional Care*, v. 24, n. 4, p. 357-370, 2010.

ROGERS, Carl R. *On Becoming a Person*. 6th ed. São Paulo: Martins Fontes, 2009.

SIOPIS G, COLAGIURI S, ALLMAN-FARINELLI M. Effectiveness of dietetic intervention for people with type 2 diabetes: A meta-analysis. *Clin Nutr*. 2021;40(5):3114-3122. doi:10.1016/j.clnu.2020.12.009

SANTOS, A. B. (2019). Qualified listening as a humanization tool for mental health care in Primary Care. *APS EM REVISTA*, 1(2), 170–179. https://doi.org/10.14295/aps.v1i2.23

SEVERINO, Ana Laura et al. Perceptions of health students on collaborative interprofessional practice in the care of patients with chronic diseases. *Physis: Revista de Saúde Coletiva*, v. 35, n. 3, 2025. DOI: 10.1590/S0103-73312025350308pt.

Chapter 15

BRAZIL. National Supplemental Health Agency (ANS). *Open Health Brasil*. [Data interoperability initiative]. Brasília: ANS. Available at: https://www.gov.br/saude/pt-br/assuntos/noticias/2022/dezembro/open-health-ministerio-da-saude-atua-para-otimizar-servicos-de-saude-no-brasil

BRAZIL. Ministry of Health. *National Humanization Policy (PNH) - Expanded and Shared Clinic*. Brasília: Ministry of Health, 2009.

BRAZIL. Ministry of Health. *National Pharmaceutical Assistance Management System (HÓRUS)*. Brasília: Ministry of Health. Available at: https://www.gov.br/saude/pt-br/composicao/sctie/daf/horus

BRAZIL. Ministry of Health. *Psychosocial Care Centers (CAPS)*. Brasília: Ministry of Health. Available at: https://www.gov.br/saude/pt-br/assuntos/saude-de-a-a-z/s/saude-mental/caps

EHEALTH ESTONIA. *The Estonian Health Information System*. Tallinn, EST. Available at: https://e-estonia.com

HAYES, Steven C.; SMITH, Spencer. *Get Out of Your Mind and Into Your Life: The New Acceptance and Commitment Therapy*. Novo Hamburgo: Sinopsys, 2022. (trans. from orig. ed. 2005).

HOOD, Leroy; FRIEND, Stephen H. Predictive, personalized, preventive, participatory (P4) cancer medicine. *Nature Reviews Clinical Oncology*, v. 8, n. 3, p. 184-187, 2011.

INSTITUTE FOR FUNCTIONAL MEDICINE (IFM). Institutional Page. Federal Way, USA. Available at: https://www.ifm.org

NEFF, Kristin. *Self-Compassion: The Proven Power of Being Kind to Yourself*. Rio de Janeiro: Sextante, 2022. (Original title: *Self-Compassion: The Proven Power of Being Kind to Yourself*).

WORLD HEALTH ORGANIZATION (WHO). *Integrated care for older people (ICOPE): guidance for person-centred assessment and pathways in primary care*. Geneva: WHO, 2024. Available at: https://www.who.int/publications/i/item/9789240103726

WORLD HEALTH ORGANIZATION (WHO). *One Health*. Geneva: WHO. Available at: https://www.who.int/health-topics/one-health

WORLD HEALTH ORGANIZATION (WHO). *The Helsinki Statement on Health in All Policies*. 8th Global Conference on Health Promotion. Helsinki, FIN: WHO, 2013. Available at: https://dssbr.ensp.fiocruz.br/wp-content/uploads/2020/11/Declara%C3%A7%C3%A3o_de_Helsinque.pdf

RIO DE JANEIRO CITY HALL. *Family Clinic*. Rio de Janeiro, BRA. Available at: https://saude.prefeitura.rio/clinica-da-familia/

SCHWARTZ, Richard C.; SWEEZY, Martha. *Internal Family Systems Therapy*. São Paulo: Roca, 2021. (Original title: *Internal Family Systems Therapy*).

SUNDHED.DK. *The Danish Public Health Portal*. Copenhagen, DEN. Available at: https://www.sundhed.dk

www.ingramcontent.com/pod-product-compliance
Lightning Source LLC
Chambersburg PA
CBHW031339230926
51848CB00002B/299
9786501649184